Advances in Cancer Immunotherapy

Edited by Shin Mukai

Published in London, United Kingdom

Advances in Cancer Immunotherapy
http://dx.doi.org/10.5772/intechopen.1001680
Edited by Shin Mukai

Contributors
Alba Mendis, Alesha Bishop, Amirhossein Ahmadieh-Yazdi, Angela Song, Dan Liu, Elycia Monaghan, Fujia Guo, Hamed Manoochehri, Hamid Tanzadehpanah, Hanie Mahaki, Hannah Shortreed, Jiachen Wen, Kuangyi Zhou, Lili Yang, Malianna Bahar Jazari, Maryam Sahlolbei, Mohadeseh Rostamipoor, Mohsen Sheykhhasan, Naser Kalhor, Niels Dawson, Nikita Trivedi, Olexiy Aseyev, Sasha Semaan, Shenglin Luan, Shin Mukai, Tianxiang Zhang, Tigran Sahakyan, Truman Ma, Tyler Halladay, Yan-Ruide Li, Yue Sun, Yuning Chen

First published in London, United Kingdom, 2024 by IntechOpen
IntechOpen is the global imprint of INTECHOPEN LIMITED, registered in England and Wales, registration number: 11086078, 167-169 Great Portland Street, London, W1W 5PF, United Kingdom

British Library Cataloguing-in-Publication Data
A catalogue record for this book is available from the British Library

Additional hard and PDF copies can be obtained from orders@intechopen.com

Advances in Cancer Immunotherapy
Edited by Shin Mukai
p. cm.
Print ISBN 978-0-85466-380-4
Online ISBN 978-0-85466-379-8
eBook (PDF) ISBN 978-0-85466-381-1

For EU product safety concerns:
IN TECH d.o.o., Prolaz Marije Krucifikse Kozulić 3, 51000 Rijeka, Croatia,
info@intechopen.com or visit our website at intechopen.com.

Meet the editor

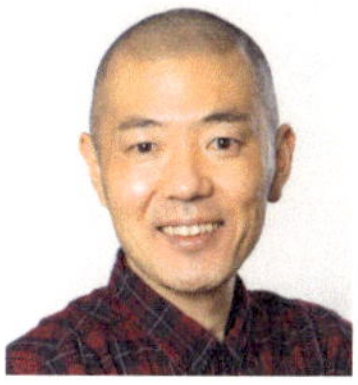

Dr. Shin Mukai is a trailblazing chemical biologist with a wealth of international experience and achievements. He completed his bachelor's and master's degrees in chemistry at Kyoto University. He obtained a Ph.D. in bio-organic chemistry at the University of Western Australia. During his first postdoctoral assignment at the Keio University School of Medicine, he developed a patented treatment of chronic graft-versus-host disease. He then moved to Boston for his second postdoctoral position at Brigham and Women's Hospital/Harvard Medical School and worked on macrophage heterogeneity. With his unique blend of expertise in synthetic organic/medicinal chemistry and biology/immunology, he co-founded the oncology pharmaceutical company New Wind Therapeutics L3C in the United States as chief executive officer and chief scientific officer in 2023.

Contents

Preface

Modern oncology places great emphasis on cancer immunotherapy, which leverages the body's immune system to combat cancer. Significant progress has been made in understanding the complex interactions between cancer cells and the immune system, leading to novel immunotherapeutic treatments.

The book *Advances in Cancer Immunotherapy* covers groundbreaking studies and the latest developments in cancer immunotherapy. It comprises seven chapters that thoroughly address different facets of cancer immunotherapy, ranging from basic principles to new therapies and clinical challenges.

Chapter 1 provides a succinct overview of the evolution of cancer immunotherapy, with a particular emphasis on the immunotherapeutic treatments approved by the United States Food and Drug Administration (FDA).

In Chapter 2, the focus is on molecular techniques to produce engineered leukocytes and the application of the engineered immune cells to the treatment of cancer.

Chapter 3 focuses on the unique characteristics of the tumor microenvironment (TME) and the strategies to target immunosuppressive components in TME for the improvement of cancer treatments.

Chapter 4 focuses on the blockade of colony-stimulating factor 1 receptor (CSF1R) as a promising approach to target tumor-associate macrophages and provides an in-depth view of the research on CSF1R inhibition and its potential therapeutic benefits.

Chapter 5 highlights the progress in chimeric antigen receptor (CAR) T-cell therapy, showcasing its development and ongoing improvements that are transforming cancer treatment.

Chapter 6 addresses the endocrine adverse events associated with cancer immunotherapy, providing insights into the underlying mechanisms and clinical strategies to mitigate these side effects.

Chapter 7 focuses on natural killer (NK) cell-based therapies, discussing the latest advancements and challenges in the use of NK cells for adoptive cell therapy against cancer.

As the editor of this book, I extend my heartfelt thanks to the distinguished contributors whose expertise has greatly enriched this volume. I hope *Advances in Cancer Immunotherapy* will be a valuable resource for researchers and clinicians, inspiring ongoing efforts to develop innovative cancer immunotherapy strategies.

Dr. Shin Mukai, Ph.D.
New Wind Therapeutics L3C,
Boston, USA

Chapter 1

Introductory Chapter: Overview of Cancer Immunotherapy

Shin Mukai

1. Introduction

Cancer is characterized by uncontrolled cell growth, and its diverse forms affect various organs and tissues, posing a significant global health threat [1, 2]. Cancer immunotherapy is a revolutionary approach and has created a paradigm shift in cancer treatment, offering hope to cancer patients [3]. Cancer immunotherapy enhances an immune response against cancer cells and is one of the most promising strategies to treat various cancer types [4]. A number of preclinical and clinical studies are ongoing, and there are a variety of efficacious immunotherapeutic modalities in cancer therapy [5]. This introductory chapter succinctly summarizes the development of cancer immunotherapy by focusing mainly on the United States Food and Drug Administration (FDA)—approved immunotherapeutic modalities.

2. Checkpoint inhibitors

Checkpoint inhibitors can remove the brakes on the immune system by preventing checkpoint ligands from binding to their receptors, leading to the effective identification and elimination of cancer cells [6]. The interaction between programmed cell death protein 1 (PD-1) on T-cells and programmed cell death ligand 1 (PD-L1) on cancer cells prevents the activation of T-cells and the induction of immune response [7]. Indeed, the blockade of PD-1/PD-L1 interaction is shown to be an effective therapeutic modality for cancer [7]. Nivolumab, Pembrolizumab, and Cemiplimab are therapeutic monoclonal antibodies that target PD-1, and FDA approved these monoclonal antibodies to treat a variety of cancer types (**Table 1**) [8–10]. Atezolizumab, Durvalumab, and Avelumab are FDA-approved monoclonal antibodies that target PD-L1 to treat several cancer types [11–13] (**Table 1**). Cytotoxic T-lymphocyte-associated protein 4 (CTLA-4) is another well-studied immune-checkpoint receptor that is expressed mainly on T-cells and represses T-cell activation [14]. As with PD-1/PD-L1 interaction, evidence suggests that the inhibition of CTLA-4 is an efficacious cancer treatment [15]. The monoclonal antibodies, Ipilimumab and Tremelimumab that target CTLA-4, received FDA approval for the treatment of several cancer types (**Table 1**) [16, 17]. Lymphocyte-activation gene 3 (LAG-3), which negatively regulates T-cell function, has emerged as the third immune-checkpoint receptor [18]. The LAG-3 blocking monoclonal antibody Relatlimab in combination with Nivolumab has received approval from FDA for the treatment of melanoma (**Table 1**) [19]. Recently, the immune regulatory protein V-domain immunoglobulin suppressor of T-cell activation (VISTA) has captured attention from research scientists [20]. VISTA is

IntechOpen

Type of immunotherapy	Drug	Targets	Indications
Checkpoint inhibitors	Nivolumab	PD-1	Melanoma
			Lung cancer
			Renal cell carcinoma
			Hodgkin lymphoma
			Head and neck cancer
			Locally advanced or metastatic urothelial carcinoma
			Metastatic colorectal cancer
			Hepatocellular carcinoma
			Advanced esophageal squamous cell carcinoma
			Esophageal or gastroesophageal junction cancer
			High-risk urothelial carcinoma
	Pembrolizumab	PD-1	Melanoma
			Lung cancer
			Head and neck squamous cell carcinoma
			Classical Hodgkin lymphoma
			Urothelial carcinoma
			Gastric or gastroesophageal junction cancer
			Cervical cancer
			Primary mediastinal large B-cell lymphoma
			Hepatocellular carcinoma
			Merkel cell carcinoma
			Esophageal squamous cell carcinoma
			Endometrial carcinoma
			Bladder cancer
			Cutaneous squamous cell carcinoma
			Colorectal cancer
			Breast cancer
			Biliary tract cancer
	Cemiplimab	PD-1	Lung cancer
			Cutaneous squamous cell carcinoma
			Basal cell carcinoma
	Atezolizumab	PD-L1	Lung cancer
			Urothelial Carcinoma
			Bladder cancer

Type of immunotherapy	Drug	Targets	Indications
			Breast cancer
			Hepatocellular carcinoma
			Melanoma
			Alveolar soft part sarcoma
	Durvalumab	PD-L1	Bladder cancer
			Lung cancer
			Biliary tract cancer
	Avelumab	PD-L1	Merkel cell carcinoma
			Urothelial carcinoma
			Renal cell carcinoma
	Ipilimumab	CTLA-4	Melanoma
			Renal cell carcinoma
			Colorectal cancer
			Hepatocellular carcinoma
			Lung cancer
			Malignant pleural mesothelioma
	Tremelimumab	CTLA-4	Hepatocellular carcinoma
			Lung cancer
	Nivolumab + Ipilimumab	PD-1 + CTLA-4	Melanoma
			Renal cell carcinoma
			Metastatic colorectal cancer
			Hepatocellular carcinoma
			Malignant pleural mesothelioma
	Nivolumab + Relatlimab	PD-1 + LAG-3	Melanoma
CAR-T therapy	Tisagenlecleucel		Acute lymphoblastic leukemia
			Large B-cell lymphoma
			Refractory follicular lymphoma
	Axicabtagene ciloleucel		Large B-cell lymphoma
			Refractory Follicular Lymphoma
	Brexucabtagene autoleucel		Mantle cell lymphoma
			B-cell acute lymphoblastic leukemia
	Lisocabtagene maraleucel		Large B-cell lymphoma
	Idecabtagene vicleucel		Multiple myeloma
	Ciltacabtegene autoleucel		Multiple myeloma

Type of immunotherapy	Drug	Targets	Indications
Cancer vaccine (preventative)	Cervarix®		Anal cancer
			Cervical cancer
			Head and neck cancer
			Penile cancer
			Vulvar cancer
			Vaginal cancer
	Gardasil®		Anal cancer
			Cervical cancer
			Head and neck cancer
			Penile cancer
			Vulvar cancer
			Vaginal cancer
	Gardasil-9®		Anal cancer
			Cervical cancer
			Head and neck cancer
			Penile cancer
			Throat cancer
			Vulvar cancer
			Vaginal cancer
	HEPLISAV-B®		Liver cancer
Cancer vaccine (therapeutic)	Bacillus Calmette-Guérin		Bladder cancer
	Sipuleucel-T		Prostate cancer
Oncolytic virus	Talimogene laherparepvec		Melanoma

Table 1.
List of FDA-approved cancer immunotherapies.

expressed on various immune cells, such as T-cells and tumor-associated macrophages (TAMs), and its binding partners are V-set and Ig domain-containing 3 (VSIG3) and P-selectin glycoprotein ligand 1 (PSGL-1) ligands [21]. VISTA on T-cells and TAMs contributes to immune tolerance [21], and the investigation into VISTA can potentially lead to the development of novel checkpoint inhibitors [20].

3. CAR-T therapy

CAR-T therapy undergoes the following processes: (i) the collection of T-cells from a patient, (ii) their genetic modification to express CAR molecules, (iii) their expansion and activation, and (iv) the infusion of the genetically modified cells back into the patient [22]. The CAR T-cells can be activated by binding to specific cancer cell antigens, eliminating cancer cells [23]. Evidence suggests that this one-time treatment can provide long-lasting immunological memory [24, 25]. Although CAR-T therapy reportedly causes adverse effects such as cytokine release syndrome and nervous system problems, the following CAR-T therapies received approval from FDA for the treatment of cancer: (i) Tisagenlecleucel, (ii) Axicabtagene ciloleucel, (iii) Brexucabtagene autoleucel, (iv) Lisocabtagene maraleucel, (v) Idecabtagene vicleucel, and (vi) Ciltacabtegene autoleucel (**Table 1**) [26–31]. A number of studies are in progress to refine and broaden CAR-T therapy for cancer [32].

4. NK cell therapy

NK cell therapy is a promising strategy to combat cancer [33]. NK cells are able to recognize and eliminate abnormal cells (such as cancer cells) that are not expressing major histocompatibility complex class I (MHC-I) [34]. Researchers have been striving to enhance the anti-cancer ability of NK cells by generating ex vivo expanded and differentiated non-engineered NK cells and chimeric antigen receptor (CAR) or CD16-engineered NK cells [35]. While there are no FDA-approved NK cell therapies to treat cancer, a number of pre-clinical clinical trials are underway [36].

5. Cancer vaccines

Cancer vaccines are designed to trigger an immune response to eliminate cancer cells [37]. There are two types of cancer vaccines [38]: therapeutic vaccines boost immune response against specific cancer cells and preventive vaccines target viruses associated with certain cancer types [38]. While tumor heterogeneity and immunosuppressive microenvironments are obstacles which impact cancer vaccine development, several cancer vaccines are approved by FDA (**Table 1**) [39, 40].

6. Oncolytic viruses

Oncolytic viruses represent a promising frontier in cancer immunotherapy and utilize genetically modified viruses [41]. Oncolytic viruses infect and replicate in cancer cells, resulting in cell rupture and the resultant release of tumor-associated antigens [42]. Consequently, the immune system detects these antigens and induces a robust immune response against infected and non-infected cancer cells [42]. This approach can boost the body's natural ability to combat cancer cells while eliminating cancer cells [43]. Of note, Talimogene laherparepvec (T-VEC), a herpes-based oncolytic virus, received approval from FDA for the treatment of melanoma (**Table 1**) [44].

7. Conclusion

Cancer immunotherapy has contributed to the advances in the field of cancer research. It should be noted that while cancer immunotherapy has offered increased treatment options and hope for cancer patients, it can cause immune-related side effects and should be carefully monitored by healthcare professionals. In order to overcome these setbacks and facilitate the development of cancer immunotherapy, artificial intelligence/machine learning (AI/ML) may be applicable for the prediction of outcomes and the optimization of therapeutic strategies.

Author details

Shin Mukai
New Wind Therapeutics L3C, Boston, United States of America

*Address all correspondence to: shin.mukai@newwindl3c.com

References

[1] Otto T, Sicinski P. Cell cycle proteins as promising targets in cancer therapy. Nature Reviews Cancer. 2017;**17**:93-115. DOI: 10.1038/nrc.2016.138

[2] Mukai S. Therapeutic approaches targeting cancer stem cells. In: Possibilities and Limitations in Current Translational Stem Cell Research. London, UK: IntechOpen; 2022. DOI: 10.5772/intechopen.108963

[3] Sambi M, Bagheri L, Szewczuk MR. Current challenges in cancer immunotherapy: Multimodal approaches to improve efficacy and patient response rates. Journal of Oncology. 2019: 4508794. DOI: 10.1155/2019/4508794

[4] Sahu M, Suryawanshi H. Immunotherapy The future of cancer treatment. Journal of Oral and Maxillofacial Pathology. 2021;**25**:371. DOI: 10.4103/0973-029X.325257

[5] Koustas E, Trifylli E-M, Sarantis P, Papadopoulos N, Karapedi E, Aloizos G, et al. Immunotherapy as a therapeutic strategy for gastrointestinal cancer-current treatment options and future perspectives. International Journal of Molecular Sciences. 2022;**23**:6664. DOI: 10.3390/ijms23126664

[6] Immune checkpoint inhibitors and their side effects. Available from: https://www.cancer.org/cancer/managing-cancer/treatment-types/immunotherapy/immune-checkpoint-inhibitors.html

[7] Alsaab HO, Sau S, Alzhrani R, Tatiparti K, Bhise K, Kashaw SK, et al. PD-1 and PD-L1 checkpoint signaling inhibition for cancer immunotherapy mechanism, combinations, and clinical outcome. Frontiers in Pharmacology. 2017;**23**:561. DOI: 10.3389/fphar.2017.00561

[8] Opdivo (Nivolumab) FDA Approval History. Available from: https://www.drugs.com/history/opdivo.html

[9] Keytruda (pembrolizumab) FDA Approval History. Available from: https://www.drugs.com/history/keytruda.html

[10] Libtayo (cemiplimab-rwlc) FDA Approval History. Available from: https://www.drugs.com/history/libtayo.html

[11] Tecentriq (atezolizumab) FDA Approval History. Available from: https://www.drugs.com/history/tecentriq.html

[12] Imfinzi (durvalumab) FDA Approval History. Available from: https://www.drugs.com/history/imfinzi.html

[13] Bavencio (avelumab) FDA Approval History. Available from: https://www.drugs.com/history/bavencio.html

[14] Tivol EA, Borriello F, Schweitzer AN, Lynch WP, Bluestone JA, Sharpe AH. Loss of CTLA-4 leads to massive lymphoproliferation and fatal multiorgan tissue destruction, revealing a critical negative regulatory role of CTLA-4. Immunity. 1995;**3**:541-547. DOI: 10.1016/1074-7613(95)90125-6

[15] Witt K, Evans-Axelsson S, Lundqvist A, Johansson M, Bjartell A, Hellsten R. Inhibition of STAT3 augments antitumor efficacy of anti-CTLA-4 treatment against prostate cancer. Cancer Immunology, Immunotherapy. 2021;**70**:3155-3166. DOI: 10.1007/s00262-021-02915-6

[16] Yervoy (ipilimumab) FDA Approval History. Available from: https://www.drugs.com/history/yervoy.html

[17] Imjudo (tremelimumab-actl) FDA Approval History. Available from: https://www.drugs.com/history/imjudo.html

[18] Triebel F, Jitsukawa S, Baixeras E, Roman-Roman S, Genevee C, Viegas-Pequignot E, et al. LAG-3, a novel lymphocyte activation gene closely related to CD4. Journal of Experimental Medicine. 1990;**171**:1393-1405. DOI: 10.1084/jem.171.5.1393

[19] Opdualag (nivolumab and relatlimab) FDA Approval History. Available from: https://www.drugs.com/history/opdualag.html

[20] Wu C, Cao X, Zhang X. VISTA inhibitors in cancer immunotherapy a short perspective on recent progresses. RSC Medicinal Chemistry. 2021;**12**: 1672-1679. DOI: 10.1039/d1md00185j

[21] Yuan L, Tatineni J, Mahoney KM, Freeman GJ. VISTA A mediator of quiescence and a promising target in cancer immunotherapy. Trends in Immunology. 2021;**42**:209-227. DOI: 10.1016/j.it.2020.12.008

[22] CAR T-Cell therapy. Available from: https://my.clevelandclinic.org/health/treatments/17726-car-t-cell-therapy

[23] Sterner RC, Sterner RM. CAR-T cell therapy current limitations and potential strategies. Blood Cancer Journal. 2021;**11**: 69. DOI: 10.1038/s41408-021-00459-7

[24] Melenhorst JJ, Chen GM, Wang M, Porter DL, Chen C, Collins MA, et al. Decade-long leukaemia remissions with persistence of CD4(+) CAR T cells. Nature. 2022;**602**:503-509. DOI: 10.1038/s41586-021-04390-6

[25] Cappell KM, Sherry RM, Yang JC, Goff SL, Vanasse DA, McIntyre L, et al. Long-term follow-up of anti-CD19 chimeric antigen receptor T-cell therapy. Journal of Clinical Oncology. 2020;**38**: 3805-3815. DOI: 10.1200/JCO.20.01467

[26] Kymriah (tisagenlecleucel) FDA Approval History. Available from: https://www.drugs.com/history/kymriah.html

[27] Yescarta (axicabtagene ciloleucel) FDA Approval History. Available from: https://www.drugs.com/history/yescarta.html

[28] Tecartus (brexucabtagene autoleucel) FDA Approval History. Available from: https://www.drugs.com/history/tecartus.html

[29] Breyanzi (lisocabtagene maraleucel) FDA Approval History. Available from: https://www.drugs.com/history/breyanzi.html

[30] Abecma (idecabtagene vicleucel) FDA Approval History. Available from: https://www.drugs.com/history/abecma.html

[31] Carvykti (ciltacabtagene autoleucel) FDA Approval History. Available from: https://www.drugs.com/history/carvykti.html

[32] CAR T-cell therapy and its side effects. Available from: https://www.cancer.org/cancer/managing-cancer/treatment-types/immunotherapy/car-t-cell1.html

[33] Chu J, Gao F, Yan M, Zhao S, Yan Z, Shi B, et al. Natural killer cells a promising immunotherapy for cancer. Journal of Translational Medicine. 2022; **20**:240. DOI: 10.1186/s12967-022-03437-0

[34] Ljunggren HG, Kärre K. In search of the 'missing self': MHC molecules and NK cell recognition. Immunology Today. 1990;**11**:237-244. DOI: 10.1016/0167-5699(90)90097-s

[35] Liu S, Galat V, Galat Y, Lee YKA, Wainwright D, Wu J. NK cell-based cancer immunotherapy from basic biology to clinical development. Journal of Hematology and Oncology. 2021;**14**:7. DOI: 10.1186/s13045-020-01014-w

[36] Lamers N, Panella D, Georgoudaki A-M, Liu H, Özkazanc D, Kučerová L, et al. Natural killer cells in clinical development as non-engineered, engineered, and combination therapies. Journal of Hematology and Oncology. 2022;**15**:164. DOI: 10.1186/s13045-022-01382-5

[37] Sellars MC, Wu CJ, Fritsch EF. Cancer vaccines: Building a bridge over troubled waters. Cell. 2022;**185**:2770-2788. DOI: 10.1016/j.cell.2022.06.035

[38] Cancer vaccines. Available from: https://www.cancercenter.com/treatment-options/precision-medicine/immunotherapy/vaccines

[39] DeMaria PJ, Bilusic M. Cancer vaccines. Hematology/Oncology Clinics of North America. 2001;**15**:741-773. DOI: 10.1016/s0889-8588(05)70245-8

[40] Cancer vaccines: Preventive, therapeutic, personalized. Available from: https://www.cancerresearch.org/treatment-types/cancer-vaccines

[41] Cristi F, Gutiérrez T, Hitt MM, Shmulevitz M. Genetic modifications that expand oncolytic virus potency. Frontiers in Molecular Biosciences. 2022;**26**:831091. DOI: 10.3389/fmolb.2022.831091

[42] Oncolytic virus enables the immune system to attack tumors. Available from: https://www.cancer.gov/news-events/cancer-currents-blog/2023/oncolytic-virus-blocking-tgf-beta

[43] Kaufman HL, Kohlhapp FJ, Zloza A. Oncolytic viruses: a new class of immunotherapy drugs. Nature Reviews Drug Discovery. 2015;**15**:660. DOI: 10.1038/nrd.2016.178

[44] Oncolytic viruses. Available from: https://cancerquest.org/patients/treatments/oncolytic-viruses?gclid=CjwKCAiAvoqsBhB9EiwA9XTWGV4YJU-FDuRtm6bm0wA9b94xgwOkFMH1lf3xDit3wxqQ3hlNc_a-fBoCsT4QAvD_BwE

Chapter 2

Engineered Cellular Immunotherapy for Cancer

Nikita Trivedi

Abstract

Cancer is the leading cause of death, accounting for nearly 1 in 6 deaths globally. Surgical removal of tumors, radiation therapy, chemotherapy, small molecular inhibitors, and tumor-specific antibodies are standard treatments for cancer. However, these treatments can have adverse off-target effects and poor tumor penetrance and can be inefficient in control and prevention of cancer. In the past several years, cell-based immunotherapies have been developed and applied in the clinic. These cell-based therapies are engineered to be tumor-specific, persistent and have reduced off-target complications. For cell-based immunotherapy, patient-derived leukocytes are harvested, manipulated *ex vivo*, and reintroduced into patients for treatment. This chapter will describe the molecular techniques used to generate engineered leukocytes, such as T cells, natural killer (NK) cells, and dendritic cells (DCs) and their applications in cancer immunotherapy.

Keywords: genome engineering, CAR T cells, NK cells, dendritic cells, PD-1/PD-L1, adoptive cell therapies, cancer immunotherapy

1. Introduction

According to the National Cancer Institute statistics, 40 percent of adults have been diagnosed with cancer at least once in their lives [1]. Surgery, radiation, and chemotherapy are major treatment strategies for cancer [2]. Over the past several years, tumor-specific cell-based therapies have been developed and have demonstrated efficacy in the clinic [3–7]. This chapter will focus on the molecular methods used to *ex vivo* manipulate immune cells and the application and effectiveness of engineered leukocytes as cancer therapeutics.

2. *Ex vivo* manipulation of patient-derived cells for cancer immunotherapy

Patient leukocytes can be derived from the peripheral blood mononuclear cells (PBMCs), cord blood cells, induced pluripotent stem cells (iPSCs), and hematopoietic stem and progenitor cells (HSPCs) [5–7]. The cells are subjected to at least one or more of the following manipulations in a laboratory: (1) induced expression of one or

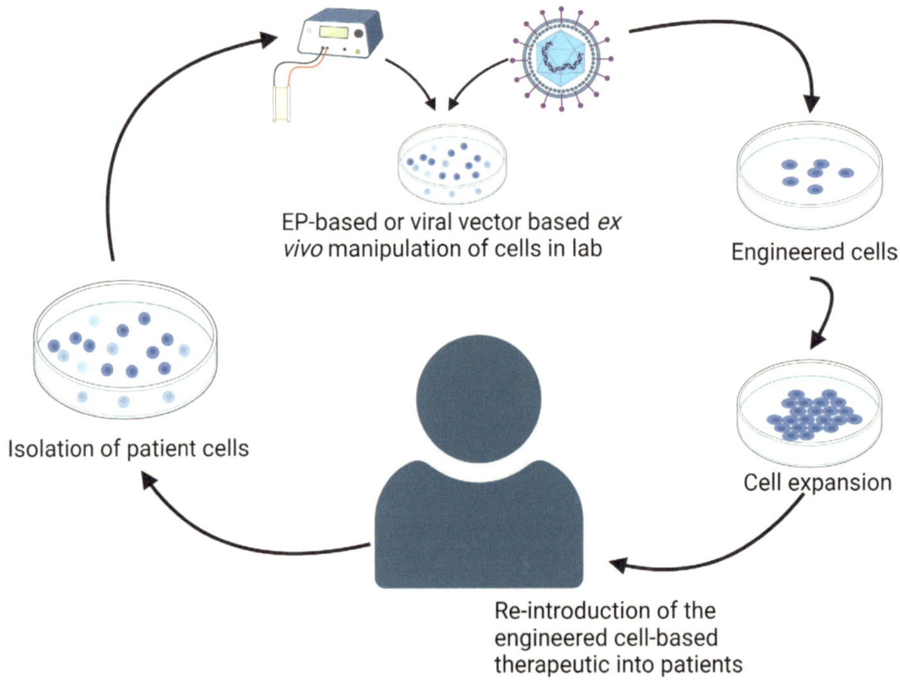

Figure 1.
Schematic demonstrating ex vivo manipulation of patient-derived cells for generating cell-based therapeutics.

more exogenous genes that confer anti-cancer properties to the cells, (2) gene knockdown or knockout to increase the efficacy of the cell therapy in evoking an immune response to the cancer, (3) exposure to factors and cytokines that expand and differentiate the donor cells into an effector population with potent anti-cancer capabilities, (4) exposure to tumor-associated antigens (TAAs) to generate an effector population capable of evoking anti-tumor immune responses [3–7]. These *ex vivo*-manipulated cells are then reintroduced into patients as autologous cell-based therapeutics [3–7]. Alternately, allogeneic engineered cells from a different donor can be introduced into cancer patients for treatment [7]. During the process of generating the anti-cancer therapeutic, the cells are subjected to several molecular methods (**Figure 1**).

3. Methods for engineering leukocytes

Ex vivo engineering of leukocytes is performed by the efficient transfer of ribonucleic acid (RNA) and deoxyribonucleic acid (DNA) cargo molecules into the cells [8]. This involves electroporation (EP), or viral vector-mediated delivery of genome editing reagents into the cells, or a combination of both techniques [8].

3.1 Molecular events of EP

EP is the application of external electric fields to cause reversible permeabilization of a cell membrane for the purpose of introducing molecules into the cell that are otherwise impermeable [9]. Patient or donor-derived cells are manipulated in a laboratory *via* EP-based transfer of RNA and DNA to induce gene disruption or exogenous gene expression. While EP is often used in the transfer of small RNA, DNA, and endonuclease enzymes into cells, its use in the transfer of large DNA vectors has been limited to a few studies because of its low efficiency [10, 11]. Large DNA constructs can be efficiently transferred by means of viral vectors [12].

3.2 mRNA-mediated gene expression

EP of messenger RNA (mRNA) is a method of gene transfer that induces transient expression of the gene of interest in the targeted cells. The mRNA is generated from a linear DNA template in a laboratory by a process known as *in vitro* transcription [13, 14]. RNA polymerase is used to generate a single-stranded mRNA transcript from a complementary DNA template [13, 14]. The mRNA undergoes several modifications to resemble a mature mRNA formed in eukaryotic cells [13, 14]. Post-transcription mRNA has a 5′ triphosphate, which is highly immunogenic [13, 14]. So, an inverted 7-methyl guanosine or 5' cap gets added [13, 14]. The 5' cap is crucial for the initiation of protein translation [13, 14]. mRNA is subject to degradation by RNA exonucleases. The addition of a polyA tail reduces mRNA degradation and increases its stability [13, 14]. The 3′ untranslated region (UTR) preceding the polyA tail has also been shown to enhance the stability of the mRNA (**Figure 2**) [13, 14].

The synthetic mRNA can be delivered to the cells as naked mRNA, or as nanoparticle formulations, or *via* EP [14]. Upon entry into the cell, translation occurs in the cytosol, and the resulting proteins structurally and functionally resemble cellular proteins [15]. The synthetic mRNA eventually undergoes degradation, and the translation of the exogenous gene halts [15]. The transient and non-integrative nature of mRNA is a crucial safety feature of mRNA therapeutics [15].

3.3 Endonucleases for gene editing

While mRNA delivery can be used for inducing transient gene expression, gene disruption and long-term expression of foreign genes can be carried out by genome editing [16]. Genome editing refers to modifications in the DNA sequence of a cell's genome in a targeted and efficient manner [16]. The two major gene editing nucleases that have been developed are zinc finger nucleases (ZFNs) and transcription activator-like effector nucleases (TALENs) [16]. The delivery of these endonucleases to the

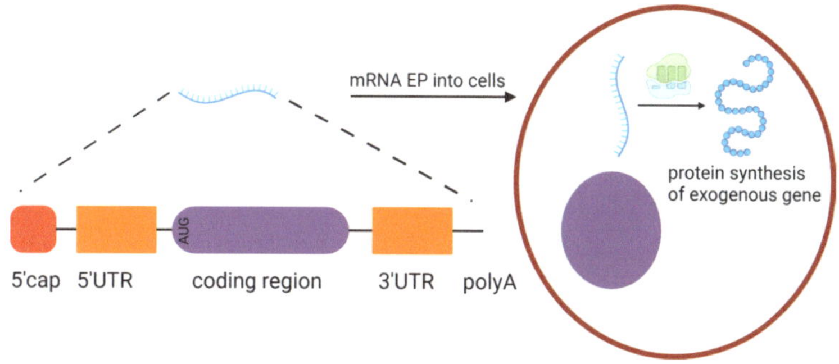

Figure 2.
Gene expression via mRNA EP. Single stranded mRNA generated by in vitro transcription consists of 5′cap, 5′UTR, coding region, 3′UTR, and a polyA tail. Upon EP into the cells, the mRNA gets translated by host machinery to form functional proteins.

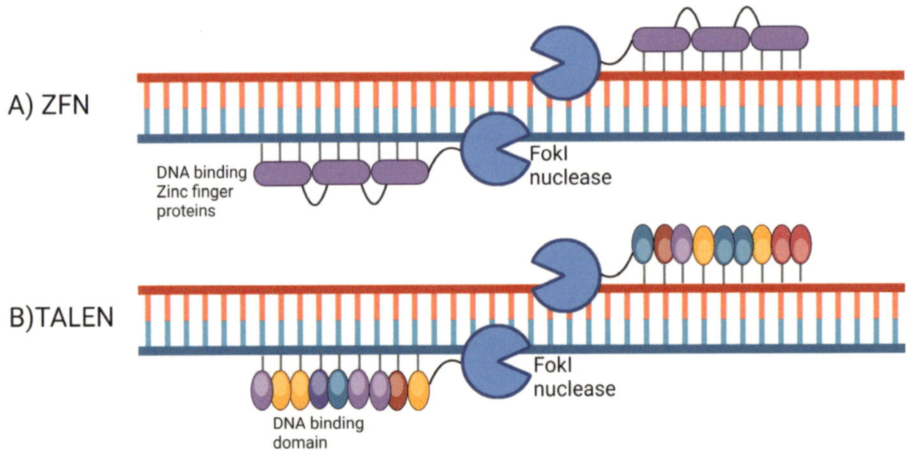

Figure 3.
Molecular mechanisms of gene editing nuclease. ZFN and TALEN consist of DNA binding proteins and FokI endonuclease. The FokI nuclease must form a dimer to make a site-specific cleavage of the target DNA.

cells can be carried out *via* EP, although direct delivery and delivery *via* viral vectors have also been tested in various studies (**Figure 3**) [17, 18].

ZFNs are chimeric proteins that constitute three to five zinc finger DNA-binding domains and a FokI endonuclease domain [19, 20]. The DNA-binding zinc finger domains are derived from transcription factors (TFs) [19, 20]. The DNA-binding domains are approximately 30 amino acids long, and they bind to three bases on the DNA [19, 20]. At least three consecutive DNA-binding domains are required for sufficient recognition [19, 20]. Two ZFNs are used to cut a single site, which is facilitated by the dimerization of the nuclease domains [21–23]. The ZFN monomer is not active until the two ZFNs assemble at the target site and form a dimer [21–23].

TALENs are proteins that are made up of DNA-binding modules linked to a FokI endonuclease cleavage domain [24]. The TALE DNA-binding repeat modules are derived from TALEs encoded by *Xanthomonas* proteobacteria [25]. The DNA-binding modules are made up of tandem repeats of approximately 34 amino acids in length [26, 27]. Like ZFNs, TALENs require dimerization of the endonuclease domain for cleavage of the target site [24].

ZFNs and TALENs are useful tools for the site-specific cleavage of DNA [21–25]. However, these techniques require expertise in protein biochemistry to generate the DNA-binding proteins for every new target site [21–25]. In comparison, clustered regularly interspaced short palindromic repeats (CRISPR)- CRISPR-associated protein 9 (Cas9) emerged as a simpler and more efficient tool for genome editing [17, 28].

3.4 Molecular mechanisms of CRISPR-Cas9 editing

CRISPR-Cas9 was discovered as a part of adaptive immunity in prokaryotic cells for the detection and cleavage of foreign nucleic acids [28, 29]. Since its discovery, it has been widely applied for genome editing (**Figure 4**) [12].

The CRISPR-Cas9 machinery consists of a CRISPR RNA (crRNA) with a spacer motif complementary to a target DNA sequence [28, 29]. The crRNA hybridizes with the target sequence adjacent to a protospacer adjacent motif (PAM) [28, 29]. PAM sites are made of the sequence NGG, where N represents any nucleotide [28, 29]. The crRNA

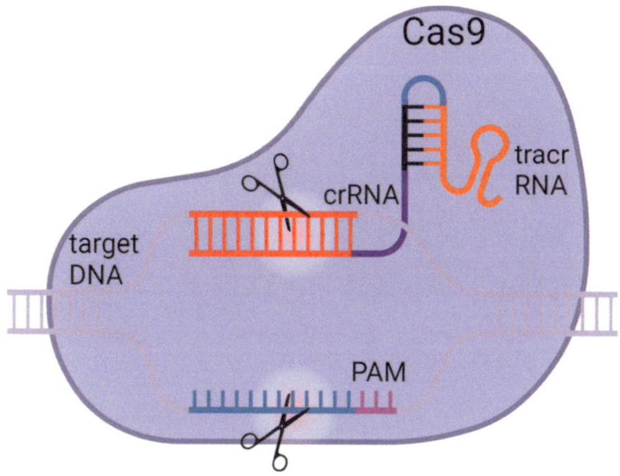

Figure 4.
CRISPR-Cas9 mediated genome editing. crRNA-tracrRNA hybrids along with the Cas9 complex are delivered to the cells via EP. Upon recognition of the target site, Cas9 nuclease makes a double stranded break in the target DNA sequence.

also hybridizes with a transactivating RNA (tracrRNA), and in turn, tracrRNA forms a complex with Cas9 [28, 29]. Alternately, single-guide RNA can also be synthesized instead of crRNA and tracrRNA hybrids [30]. The CRISPR-Cas9 complexes are delivered into the cells *via* EP [31]. Upon hybridization of the spacer motif of the crRNA to a target sequence, the Cas9 protein makes a blunt double-stranded break [28, 29]. In this method, Cas9 generates a site-specific cleavage with high efficiency [28, 29].

3.5 DNA repair pathways

Endonucleases have been used to induce double-stranded DNA breaks into the genome of cells [17, 18]. These DNA breaks trigger the DNA repair pathway in the cells. In eukaryotic cells, DNA breaks can be repaired by the error-prone process of nonhomologous end joining (NHEJ) [32]. During NHEJ, nucleotide insertions or deletions (indels) can happen at the site of the cleavage [32]. These indels can cause frame shifts or introduce premature stop codons, causing disruption in the expression of the target gene [32].

Another method of DNA repair is known as homology-directed repair (HDR). It can occur naturally in cells by using sister chromatid or can be induced experimentally by providing repair templates that are complementary to the site of DNA break [33, 34]. HDR can be used to integrate exogenous genes into the genome of a cell and drive the expression of foreign genes using the host transcription and translation machinery [35].

HDR repair templates or donor templates are either single-stranded oligodeoxynucleotides or double-stranded DNA vectors that have two homology arms with sequences complementary to the region on either side of the targeted DNA break site [36]. The 5' homology arm is followed by a promoter to drive expression of the inserted gene [37]. The promoter is adjacent to the exogenous gene, which gets inserted at the site of the double-stranded DNA break [37]. Because of the large size of the DNA repair templates, their delivery into the cells is challenging [10, 11]. In most genome editing studies, viral vectors are a preferred method for the delivery of DNA repair templates (**Figure 5**) [12].

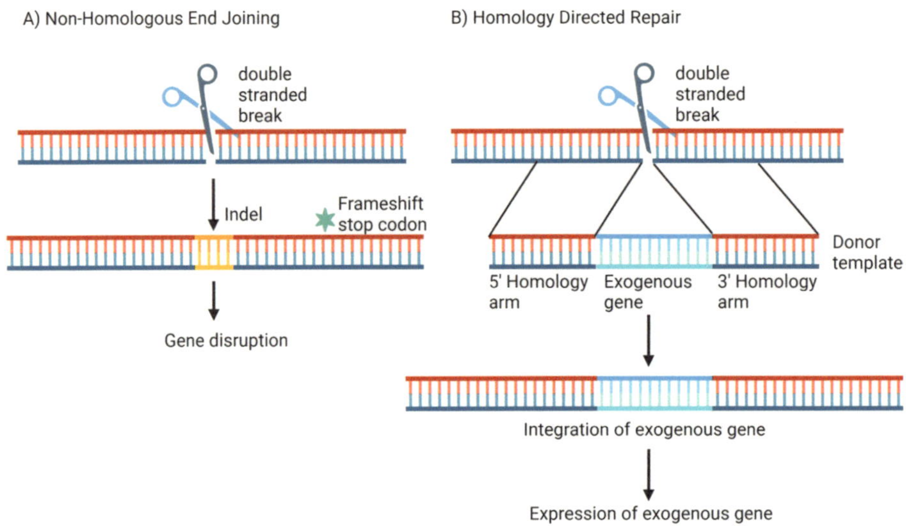

Figure 5.
DNA repair pathways following double-stranded DNA break. (A) NHEJ is error prone and it leads to indels in the sequence which can cause gene disruption. (B) HDR can be induced by providing repair templates for the expression of exogenous gene at the targeted loci.

3.6 Viral vectors for genome engineering

Following endonuclease-mediated double-stranded DNA breaks, viral vectors such as adeno-associated viral vectors can be provided as a repair template to integrate the gene of interest at the targeted location [37]. On the other hand, vectors such as lentiviral vectors do not integrate at a specific target site but instead integrate at various sites in the actively transcribed gene loci of the transduced cell [38]. The most commonly used viral vectors for *ex vivo* genome engineering of leukocytes are adenovirus vectors, adeno-associated virus vectors, retrovirus vectors, and lentivirus vectors [39]. Each viral vector has several different serotypes that demonstrate tropism to certain cell types and therefore can be used for editing specific cell types [39]. The viral vectors have specific capsid or envelope proteins that can bind to receptors on the cell surface, causing internalization of the viral vector and the delivery of the DNA cargo into the cytosol [12]. The DNA cargo migrates into the nucleus and integrates into the genome. Alternately, certain viral genomes reside episomally within the host cell [39]. These viral vectors are a means to incorporate and induce the expression of exogenous genes in donor cells (**Table 1**) [39].

4. Preclinical and clinical outcomes of engineered leukocytes in cancer immunotherapy

The advent of molecular techniques has facilitated the development of cell-based cancer immunotherapy. This section will discuss the leukocyte populations that have been engineered and are clinically relevant for cancer immunotherapy.

Method	Purpose	Advantages	Drawbacks	References
mRNA-mediated gene expression	Exogenous gene expression	High transfection efficiency Low-risk non-integrative method	Transient secretion of exogenous proteins because of low mRNA stability	[13–15]
Viral vectors	Exogenous gene expression	Long-term secretion of exogenous protein by the transduced cells Delivery of large DNA constructs at the targeted loci	Possible risk of insertional mutagenesis Cells must express surface receptors capable of binding viral vectors Potential immunogenicity from vector component	[37–39]
ZFNs and TALENs	Induce double-stranded DNA breaks	DNA-binding domains can be designed for any target site	Requires expertise in protein biochemistry to develop reagents Endonuclease requires dimerization	[21–25]
CRISPR-Cas9	Induce double-stranded DNA breaks	Simple and efficient design of guides	Target sites dependent on PAM sequences Potential off-target cuts	[28, 29, 40]

Table 1.
Comparison of different methods to engineer leukocytes.

4.1 Engineered T cells for cancer immunotherapy

Immune cells play a crucial role in providing defense against tumors by specifically targeting and killing cancer cells [41]. White blood cells known as T lymphocytes can recognize tumor-associated antigens when presented by proteins known as the Major Histocompatibility Complex (MHC) [42]. Upon recognition of the tumor-associated antigens, T cells undergo activation and release cytotoxic proteins that target the tumor cells [43]. Moreover, T cells can release inflammatory cytokines that can activate other immune cells and promote tumor clearance [43]. For efficient recognition of cancer cells, T cells have been engineered to express tumor antigen-specific T cell receptors (TCR) [44, 45]. However, tumor cells can downregulate the expression of MHC and therefore reduce the presentation of the antigens and evade immune recognition [43].

4.1.1 Chimeric antigen receptor T cells

To facilitate T cells to recognize tumor cells in the absence of MHC proteins, chimeric antigen receptor T cells (CAR T cells) were designed [46]. The CAR is a synthetic receptor that directs the T cells to recognize antigen-expressing tumor cells directly without the need for MHC proteins [46]. The CAR consists of an antigen-binding domain on the extracellular side, which is derived from antigen-binding regions of antibodies [47]. The antigen-binding domain is linked to intracellular signaling domains (for example, CD3 zeta), which induces T cell activation [47]. There are also certain co-stimulatory receptor intracellular domains that enhance signaling post-activation [47].

The CAR can be expressed *via* genomic integration using viral vectors or by the EP of CAR mRNA into the T cells [3, 4, 48–50]. These engineered CAR T cells can

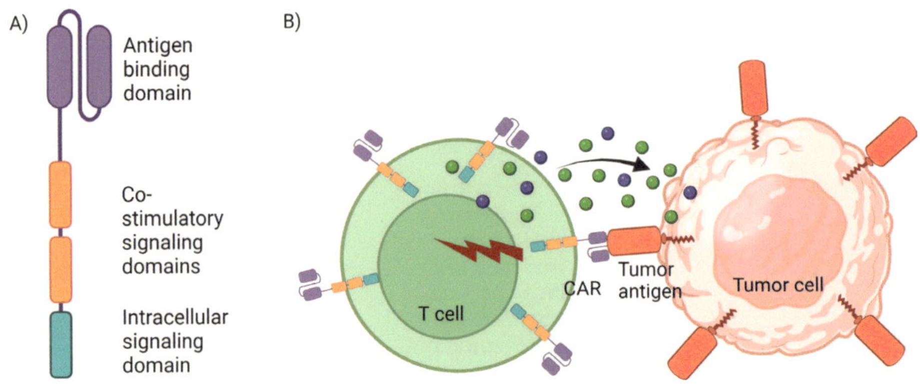

Figure 6.
CAR T cell structure and function. (A) The structure of a CAR. (B) Engineered T cell expressing CAR bind to an antigen on the surface of a tumor cell. Upon antigen recognition, CAR T cell becomes activated and releases cytokines and cytotoxic molecules to kill the tumor cell.

be reintroduced into patients as therapeutics [3, 4, 48–50]. The T lymphocytes get activated upon CAR-mediated recognition of the tumor antigen and release cytotoxic and inflammatory molecules that target the tumor cells [47]. CAR T cell therapy has shown high efficacy in the treatment of B cell malignancies (**Figure 6**) [51–54].

4.1.2 Engineered TCR-based therapeutics

Unlike hematologic malignancies, CAR T cell treatment in solid tumors has not yielded encouraging results [55]. Engineered T cell receptor therapy is an alternative to CAR T cell therapy [56]. CAR T cells are restricted to the recognition of surface antigens, whereas TCR can recognize surface and intracellular antigens presented by APCs [56]. Moreover, TCR requires a lower epitope density for activation than a CAR, which can lead to efficient T cell responses in tumors with low antigen expression [56]. Because of these reasons, engineered TCRs have been developed for the treatment of various cancers.

Engineered T cells that are specific to different cancer antigens such as melanoma antigen recognized by T cells-1 (MART-1), glycoprotein-100, carcinoembryonic antigen (CEA), cancer testis antigen called NY-ESO-1, and melanoma antigen gene protein family (MAGE) have been generated [57–61]. These engineered T cells have also been tested in clinical trials and have produced encouraging results [57–61]. For instance, in patients with metastatic synovial sarcoma, T cells engineered to express TCR specific to the cancer antigen NY-ESO-1 were infused into patients [60]. The treatment showed persistence of edited cells for about 6 months, and antitumor responses were observed in 50 percent of the patients [60]. Currently, more work is being done to find cancer neoantigens to develop neo-TCR-engineered T cells with enhanced tumor-specificity [62].

4.1.3 T cell gene disruption in cancer immunotherapy

A major challenge in the treatment of cancer is the immunosuppressive tumor microenvironment (TME). To evade detection and clearance, tumor cells express surface proteins that can suppress the immune cells [63]. One such surface protein is known as programmed death ligand 1 (PD-L1), which is highly expressed by several cancer cells [63]. PD-L1 interacts with another protein expressed on immune cells, especially T lymphocytes, known as programmed cell death protein-1 (PD-1) [63]. The PD-L1-PD-1 interaction limits T cell activation and prevents effective tumor clearance [63]. Elimination of PD-1 in T cells enhances T cell activation and the killing of cancer cells. EP of CRISPR-Cas9 or TALEN reagents have been used to disrupt the expression of the PD-1 gene in T cells [50, 64].

Recent studies in cancer immunotherapy have now focused on multiplex genome editing [3, 4]. Patient-derived T cells are harvested and are manipulated to induce the expression of a CAR or tumor antigen-specific T cell receptor along with disruption of immunosuppressive genes such as PD-1 [3, 4]. The multiplex genome editing approach allows the generation and delivery of novel cell-based therapies that are more effective than conventional cell-based therapies.

4.2 Engineered natural killer (NK) cells for cancer immunotherapy

Engineered T cells have shown efficacy in cancer immunotherapy; however, generating autologous engineered T cells is an expensive and time-consuming process [65]. NK cells can be an allogeneic donor for CAR therapy that does not cause graft versus host disease [65]. NK cells are lymphocytes that, like T cells, also have the capacity to target tumor cells through the release of cytotoxic and inflammatory molecules [66]. NK cells have multiple mechanisms to carry out tumor killing, which include activation *via* surface receptors, engineered CARs, and antibodies [66]. Upon activation, NK cells release cytotoxic granules consisting of perforin and granzyme that perforate and kill the target cells [66].

Another advantage of developing NK cells as an allogeneic therapeutic product is the source of the donor NK cells [67, 68]. NK cells can be generated from PBMCs, iPSCs, and cord blood cells [7, 67, 68]. The cord blood-derived NK cells provide a rich source that can be expanded *in vitro* by the addition of recombinant factors and cytokines [67, 68]. These *in vitro*-generated NK cells can be engineered to produce an NK-CAR product [68, 69].

4.2.1 CAR-NK therapy

Several studies have been done on the development of NK-CAR [70–72]. Activation of NK cells occur through the engagement of the surface receptor known as NKG2D [73–75]. The ligand for NKG2D is expressed on cancer cells [73–75]. NK-CAR is made up of the NKG2D receptor protein and intracellular activating domains [73–75]. The NK-CAR is delivered into NK cells *via* EP, and the NK-CAR-expressing cells are reintroduced into patients for tumor clearance [73–75].

NK cells can also be engineered to express tumor-antigen-specific CARs, similar to CAR T cells [69, 76]. Cord blood-derived NK cells expressing anti-CD19 CAR have been administered in phase 1 and 2 clinical trials for lymphoma and leukemia patients [76]. There was a 73 percent response rate among patients without the development of any adverse effects [76]. CAR-NK treatments that target the tumor antigen CD70 are being developed for non-Hodgkin lymphoma [69]. This NK cell therapy is currently being tested in a clinical trial (NCT05092451) for patients with CD70-expressing hematological malignancies [77].

Over the past several years, NK cell therapies have evolved to become long-lasting and efficacious anti-cancer therapies. Interleukin 15 was incorporated as part of the CAR construct to maintain the metabolic fitness and effector functions of the CAR

NK cells in the TME [78, 79]. In another study, an NK self-recognizing inhibitory CAR was co-expressed with a tumor-targeting activating CAR to prevent NK cells from killing sibling NK cells [79]. Both studies demonstrate that NK cell therapies can be subjected to innovative engineering to generate a persistent and efficient therapeutic product [78, 79].

4.3 Engineered dendritic cells (DCs) for cancer immunotherapy

DCs are specialized immune cells that reside in lymphoid and nonlymphoid compartments and act as sentinels [80]. Upon antigen encounter, DCs can efficiently capture antigen, process it, and present it in the context of MHCI and MHCII molecules [5, 81]. DC-mediated antigen presentation is a major pathway that facilitates the activation and expansion of antigen-specific CD4 and CD8 T cells [5, 81]. DCs also display the capacity to migrate between lymphoid and nonlymphoid tissues, causing antigen spreading [5, 81]. DCs can modulate inflammatory signals and control lymphocyte homing to various tissues [5, 81]. Because of these properties, manipulating DCs can mediate the regulation of the TME [5, 81]. For the purposes of immunotherapy, patient-derived peripheral blood monocytes or HSPCs can be treated with recombinant cytokines or factors to induce differentiation and maturation into a DC population [5, 82, 83].

4.3.1 DCs as APCs in cancer

To exploit the APC function of DCs in cancer immunotherapy, patient-derived DCs can be loaded with TAA and injected back into patients [83]. The TAA can be introduced into DCs by incubation with tumor lysates, or by incubation with tumor-derived or recombinant peptides, or *via* EP of mRNA encoding for tumor antigens into the DCs [83]. For metastatic prostate cancers, a DC-based therapy known as sipuleucel-T is approved by the Food and Drug Administration [84]. In this treatment, patient-derived immune cells are incubated with tumor antigen prostate-specific phosphatase to generate potent tumor-specific APCs that are reintroduced into patients to activate anti-tumor immune responses [84]. In ovarian cancer, incubation of patient-derived DCs with autologous whole tumor lysates demonstrated efficient generation of a DC-based vaccine [85]. Vaccination induced a T cell response against known tumor epitopes as well as previously unrecognized neoepitopes [85]. The potent T cell response against autologous tumor antigens was associated with prolonged patient survival [85]. In a phase 2 study of acute myeloid leukemia, DCs electroporated with the tumor antigen known as Wilm's tumor 1 mRNA were given as post-remission treatment [86]. This DC vaccination was demonstrated as an effective strategy to prevent or delay the chance of relapse in patients that are in remission [86]. These studies have highlighted the importance of DCs in driving a tumor antigen-specific T cell response, tumor control, and prevention.

4.3.2 Engineered DCs in the TME

DCs can also be edited to knock out certain proteins that reduce their effector functions [87–89]. Deletion of protein associated with the antigen processing pathways, such as YTHDF1, has demonstrated improved antigen presentation and anti-tumor T cell responses [89]. To enhance the immune stimulatory capacity of DCs, overexpression of proteins that increase DC effector function has been employed [87, 88]. In patients with non-small cell lung carcinoma, peripheral blood-derived DCs were transduced to express the C-C motif chemokine ligand 21 (CCL21) using an adenoviral vector [90]. Intra-tumor vaccination with CCL21-expressing DCs demonstrated a systemic increase in anti-tumor responses along with a localized increase in the infiltration of CD8 T cells in the TME [90].

These studies showcase a range of functions performed by DCs and a central role for DCs in driving antigen-specific T cell responses in cancer.

5. Limitations and future directions

Cell-based immunotherapies have revolutionized cancer treatments through the development of tumor-specific and personalized regimens for patients. However, there are several areas of cell-based cancer immunotherapy that need improvement.

5.1 Low persistence of engineered cells in patients

A major reason for the poor outcome of cell-based cancer immunotherapy is the limited persistence of the engineered T cells [91]. Recent studies have shown that a T cell memory-like transcriptomic profile of CAR T cells is associated with good treatment outcomes and the long-term persistence of cells [92]. A TF known as FOXO1 is involved in the memory programming of CAR T cells [93]. In future studies, CAR T cells with memory reprogramming can be generated to increase the persistence and efficacy of CAR T cell therapy.

5.2 Toxicity from cell-based immunotherapy

CAR T cells have been effective in hematological malignancies; however, infusion of CAR T cells has been associated with severe adverse effects [94]. Cytokine release syndrome (CRS) occurs because of systemic inflammation and a rise in the level of cytokines upon CAR T injection [94]. An antibody that blocks the interleukin-6 receptor is used as a treatment measure for CRS [94]. Patients are also at risk of developing immune effector cell-associated neurotoxicity syndrome (ICANS) and need to be in the care of a trained professional that can recognize the signs of ICANS [94]. Intensive care support and corticosteroids are used to treat ICANS [94]. These adverse effects last from hours to several days post-infusion of CAR T cells [94]. Another challenge is the application of CAR T cells in the treatment of solid tumors [95]. The CAR T cells can target nonmalignant tissue that expresses the tumor antigen and cause substantial toxicity [95]. Safe cell-based therapies with reduced systemic adverse effects need to be developed. NK cell therapies have shown efficacy in tumor control without the adverse effects associated with T cell therapies [65].

5.3 Off-the-shelf engineered cell-based therapy

Cell-based treatments are generated from autologous cells that are harvested from individual patients, manipulated *ex vivo*, and reintroduced into the same patient [3–7]. While this method ensures personalized treatment, the process of generating patient-derived engineered cells is expensive, time-consuming, labor-intensive, and requires expertise [3–7]. Also, this method is dependent on the patient having a sufficient population of donor cells. Therefore, having an alternative allogeneic cell-based product or off-the-shelf product will be cost-effective, rapid, and universally applicable to more patients [65, 69, 76]. The generation of engineered NK cells is a step in the direction of generating off-the-shelf products and should be further developed [65, 69, 76].

5.4 *In vivo* engineering of leukocytes for cancer immunotherapy

Another drawback of the current state of cell-based therapies is the duration and feasibility of *ex vivo* cell manufacturing [96, 97]. Biotechnology companies are studying ways to deliver viral vectors to engineer cells *in vivo* rather than manipulating cells *ex vivo* [96, 97]. VivoVec, a replication-incompetent lentiviral vector platform, has been developed by Umoja Biopharma to generate CAR T cells [97]. The VivoVec particle expresses an anti-CD3 single-chain variable fragment that allows it to bind and transduce T cells [97]. Upon transduction, a payload transgene consisting of anti-CD19 CAR gets expressed by the T cells [97]. Administration of VivoVec particles to humanized mice with CD19-expressing tumors demonstrated expansion of CAR T cells and clearance of B cell tumors [97]. Interius Biotherapeutics has also developed a non-replicating, self-inactivating lentiviral vector delivery platform to generate anti-CD20 CAR T cells and CAR NK cells [96]. The lentiviral vector expresses surface anti-CD7, which allows it to bind and transduce T cells and NK cells [96]. The T cells and NK cells express the functional anti-CD20 CAR, and this strategy has been shown to be efficacious in tumor clearance in preclinical models [96]. Taken together, these studies demonstrate the advances in gene therapy for cancer treatments.

6. Conclusion

Engineered leukocytes have been a major advance in cancer therapeutics because they generate tumor-specific immune responses in an autologous manner for patients. The efficacy of CAR T cells has been very encouraging for the further development of engineered leukocytes. However, the personalized treatment approach using autologous cells is expensive and not feasible to administer to a large cohort of patients. There is a need to develop allogeneic engineered products such as NK CARs that are well tolerated, efficacious, and can be applied universally to patients. Another approach that does not require donor cells is gene therapy platforms that can generate tumor-specific engineered cells *in vivo* by delivering viral vectors. However, treatment with viral vectors always presents a risk of immunogenicity and insertional mutagenesis. Overall, cell-based immunotherapies have revolutionized cancer treatments and will continue to evolve in the future.

Acknowledgements

All figures were prepared using Biorender.com.

Conflict of interest

The author declares no conflict of interest.

Acronyms and abbreviations

NK	natural killer
DCs	dendritic cells
PBMCs	peripheral blood mononuclear cells
iPSCs	induced pluripotent stem cells
HSPCs	hematopoietic stem and progenitor cells
TAA	tumor-associated antigen
RNA	ribonucleic acid
DNA	deoxyribonucleic acid
EP	electroporation
mRNA	messenger ribonucleic acid
UTR	untranslated region
ZFN	zinc finger nuclease
TALEN	transcription activator-like effector nucleases
TF	transcription factor
CRISPR	clustered regularly interspaced short palindromic repeats
Cas9	CRISPR-associated protein 9
crRNA	CRISPR RNA
PAM	protospacer adjacent motif
tracr RNA	trans-activating RNA
NHEJ	nonhomologous end joining
HDR	homology-directed repair
MHC	major histocompatibility class
TCR	T cell receptor
CAR	chimeric antigen receptor
MART-1	melanoma antigen recognized by T cells-1
CEA	colorectal cancer antigen carcinoembryonic antigen
MAGE	melanoma antigen gene protein family
TME	tumor microenvironment
PD-L1	programmed death ligand-1
PD-1	programmed cell death protein-1
CCL21	C-C motif chemokine ligand 21
CRS	cytokine release syndrome
ICANS	immune effector cell-associated neurotoxicity syndrome

Author details

Nikita Trivedi
Seattle Children's Research Institute, Seattle, United States

*Address all correspondence to: nikita.trivedi@seattlechildrens.org

References

[1] National Cancer Institute. Cancer Statistics. 2020. Available from: https://www.cancer.gov/about-cancer/understanding/statistics

[2] Saini KS, Twelves C. Determining lines of therapy in patients with solid cancers: A proposed new systematic and comprehensive framework. British Journal of Cancer. 2021;**125**(2):155-163

[3] Ren J et al. Multiplex genome editing to generate universal CAR T cells resistant to PD1 inhibition. Clinical Cancer Research. 2017;**23**(9):2255-2266

[4] Stadtmauer EA et al. CRISPR-engineered T cells in patients with refractory cancer. Science. 2020;**367**(6481):eaba7365

[5] Perez CR, De Palma M. Engineering dendritic cell vaccines to improve cancer immunotherapy. Nature Communications. 2019;**10**(1):5408

[6] Abou-El-Enein M et al. Scalable manufacturing of CAR T cells for cancer immunotherapy. Blood Cancer Discovery. 2021;**2**(5):408-422

[7] Shin MH et al. NK cell-based immunotherapies in cancer. Immune Network. 2020;**20**(2):e14

[8] Lukjanov V, Koutna I, Simara P. CAR T-cell production using nonviral approaches. Journal of Immunology Research. 2021;**2021**:6644685

[9] Kotnik T et al. Cell membrane electroporation-part 1: The phenomenon. IEEE Electrical Insulation Magazine. 2012;**28**(5):14-23

[10] Lesueur LL, Mir LM, Andre FM. Overcoming the specific toxicity of large plasmids electrotransfer in primary cells in vitro. Molecular Therapy - Nucleic Acids. 2016;**5**(3):e291

[11] Ribeiro S et al. Plasmid DNA size does affect nonviral gene delivery efficiency in stem cells. Cellular Reprogramming. 2012;**14**(2):130-137

[12] Lino CA et al. Delivering CRISPR: A review of the challenges and approaches. Drug Delivery. 2018;**25**(1):1234-1257

[13] Beck JD et al. mRNA therapeutics in cancer immunotherapy. Molecular Cancer. 2021;**20**(1):69

[14] Deng Z et al. mRNA vaccines: The dawn of a new era of cancer immunotherapy. Frontiers in Immunology. 2022;**13**:887125

[15] Qin S et al. mRNA-based therapeutics: Powerful and versatile tools to combat diseases. Signal Transduction and Targeted Therapy. 2022;**7**(1):166

[16] Shamshirgaran Y et al. Tools for efficient genome editing; ZFN, TALEN, and CRISPR. Methods in Molecular Biology. 2022;**2495**:29-46

[17] Bhardwaj A, Nain V. TALENs-an indispensable tool in the era of CRISPR: A mini review. Journal, Genetic Engineering & Biotechnology. 2021;**19**(1):125

[18] Bobis-Wozowicz S et al. Non-integrating gamma-retroviral vectors as a versatile tool for transient zinc-finger nuclease delivery. Scientific Reports. 2014;**4**:4656

[19] Carroll D. Genome engineering with zinc-finger nucleases. Genetics. 2011;**188**(4):773-782

[20] Pabo CO, Peisach E, Grant RA. Design and selection of novel Cys2His2 zinc finger proteins. Annual Review of Biochemistry. 2001;**70**:313-340

[21] Bitinaite J et al. FokI dimerization is required for DNA cleavage. Proceedings of the National Academy of Sciences of the United States of America. 1998;**95**(18):10570-10575

[22] Kim YG, Cha J, Chandrasegaran S. Hybrid restriction enzymes: Zinc finger fusions to Fok I cleavage domain. Proceedings of the National Academy of Sciences of the United States of America. 1996;**93**(3):1156-1160

[23] Smith J et al. Requirements for double-strand cleavage by chimeric restriction enzymes with zinc finger DNA-recognition domains. Nucleic Acids Research. 2000;**28**(17):3361-3369

[24] Joung JK, Sander JD. TALENs: A widely applicable technology for targeted genome editing. Nature Reviews. Molecular Cell Biology. 2013;**14**(1):49-55

[25] Bogdanove AJ, Voytas DF. TAL effectors: Customizable proteins for DNA targeting. Science. 2011;**333**(6051):1843-1846

[26] Boch J et al. Breaking the code of DNA binding specificity of TAL-type III effectors. Science. 2009;**326**(5959):1509-1512

[27] Moscou MJ, Bogdanove AJ. A simple cipher governs DNA recognition by TAL effectors. Science. 2009;**326**(5959):1501

[28] Jinek M et al. A programmable dual-RNA-guided DNA endonuclease in adaptive bacterial immunity. Science. 2012;**337**(6096):816-821

[29] Cong L et al. Multiplex genome engineering using CRISPR/Cas systems. Science. 2013;**339**(6121):819-823

[30] Chen B et al. Dynamic imaging of genomic loci in living human cells by an optimized CRISPR/Cas system. Cell. 2013;**155**(7):1479-1491

[31] Horodecka K, Duchler M. CRISPR/Cas9: Principle, applications, and delivery through extracellular vesicles. International Journal of Molecular Sciences. 2021;**22**(11):6072

[32] Lieber MR. The mechanism of double-strand DNA break repair by the nonhomologous DNA end-joining pathway. Annual Review of Biochemistry. 2010;**79**:181-211

[33] Carroll D. Genome engineering with targetable nucleases. Annual Review of Biochemistry. 2014;**83**:409-439

[34] Wang J et al. Homology-driven genome editing in hematopoietic stem and progenitor cells using ZFN mRNA and AAV6 donors. Nature Biotechnology. 2015;**33**(12):1256-1263

[35] Schubert MS et al. Optimized design parameters for CRISPR Cas9 and Cas12a homology-directed repair. Scientific Reports. 2021;**11**(1):19482

[36] Ran FA et al. Genome engineering using the CRISPR-Cas9 system. Nature Protocols. 2013;**8**(11):2281-2308

[37] Li C, Samulski RJ. Engineering adeno-associated virus vectors for gene therapy. Nature Reviews. Genetics. 2020;**21**(4):255-272

[38] Poletti V, Mavilio F. Designing lentiviral vectors for gene therapy of genetic diseases. Viruses. 2021;**13**(8):1526

[39] Bulcha JT et al. Viral vector platforms within the gene therapy landscape. Signal Transduction and Targeted Therapy. 2021;**6**(1):53

[40] Yip BH. Recent advances in CRISPR/Cas9 delivery strategies. Biomolecules. 2020;**10**(6):839

[41] Hiam-Galvez KJ, Allen BM, Spitzer MH. Systemic immunity in cancer. Nature Reviews. Cancer. 2021;**21**(6):345-359

[42] Geiger TL, Jyothi MD. Development and application of receptor-modified T lymphocytes for adoptive immunotherapy. Transfusion Medicine Reviews. 2001;**15**(1):21-34

[43] Shah K et al. T cell receptor (TCR) signaling in health and disease. Signal Transduction and Targeted Therapy. 2021;**6**(1):412

[44] Schober K et al. Orthotopic replacement of T-cell receptor alpha- and beta-chains with preservation of near-physiological T-cell function. Nature Biomedical Engineering. 2019;**3**(12):974-984

[45] Rapoport AP et al. NY-ESO-1-specific TCR-engineered T cells mediate sustained antigen-specific antitumor effects in myeloma. Nature Medicine. 2015;**21**(8):914-921

[46] Sterner RC, Sterner RM. CAR-T cell therapy: Current limitations and potential strategies. Blood Cancer Journal. 2021;**11**(4):69

[47] Jayaraman J et al. CAR-T design: Elements and their synergistic function. eBioMedicine. 2020;**58**:102931

[48] Cherkassky L et al. Human CAR T cells with cell-intrinsic PD-1 checkpoint blockade resist tumor-mediated inhibition. The Journal of Clinical Investigation. 2016;**126**(8):3130-3144

[49] Serganova I et al. Enhancement of PSMA-directed CAR adoptive immunotherapy by PD-1/PD-L1 blockade. Molecular Therapy - Oncolytics. 2017;**4**:41-54

[50] Rupp LJ et al. CRISPR/Cas9-mediated PD-1 disruption enhances anti-tumor efficacy of human chimeric antigen receptor T cells. Scientific Reports. 2017;7(1):737

[51] Brentjens RJ et al. CD19-targeted T cells rapidly induce molecular remissions in adults with chemotherapy-refractory acute lymphoblastic leukemia. Science Translational Medicine. 2013;**5**(177):177ra38

[52] Kalos M et al. T cells with chimeric antigen receptors have potent antitumor effects and can establish memory in patients with advanced leukemia. Science Translational Medicine. 2011;**3**(95):95ra73

[53] Maude SL et al. Chimeric antigen receptor T cells for sustained remissions in leukemia. The New England Journal of Medicine. 2014;**371**(16):1507-1517

[54] Turtle CJ et al. CD19 CAR-T cells of defined CD4+:CD8+ composition in adult B cell ALL patients. The Journal of Clinical Investigation. 2016;**126**(6):2123-2138

[55] Albelda SM. CAR T cell therapy for patients with solid tumours: Key lessons to learn and unlearn. Nature Reviews. Clinical Oncology. 2024;**21**(1):47-66

[56] Baulu E et al. TCR-engineered T cell therapy in solid tumors: State of the art and perspectives. Science Advances. 2023;**9**(7):eadf3700

[57] Johnson LA et al. Gene therapy with human and mouse T-cell receptors mediates cancer regression and targets normal tissues expressing cognate antigen. Blood. 2009;**114**(3):535-546

[58] Parkhurst MR et al. T cells targeting carcinoembryonic antigen can mediate regression of metastatic colorectal cancer but induce severe transient colitis. Molecular Therapy. 2011;**19**(3):620-626

[59] Robbins PF et al. A pilot trial using lymphocytes genetically engineered with an NY-ESO-1-reactive T-cell receptor: Long-term follow-up and correlates with response. Clinical Cancer Research. 2015;**21**(5):1019-1027

[60] D'Angelo SP et al. Antitumor activity associated with prolonged persistence of adoptively transferred NY-ESO-1 (c259) T cells in synovial sarcoma. Cancer Discovery. 2018;**8**(8):944-957

[61] Ramachandran I et al. Systemic and local immunity following adoptive transfer of NY-ESO-1 SPEAR T cells in synovial sarcoma. Journal for Immunotherapy of Cancer. 2019;**7**(1):276

[62] Pang Z et al. Neoantigen-targeted TCR-engineered T cell immunotherapy: Current advances and challenges. Biomarker Research. 2023;**11**(1):104

[63] Ai L, Xu A, Xu J. Roles of PD-1/PD-L1 pathway: Signaling, cancer, and beyond. Advances in Experimental Medicine and Biology. 2020;**1248**:33-59

[64] Menger L et al. TALEN-mediated inactivation of PD-1 in tumor-reactive lymphocytes promotes intratumoral T-cell persistence and rejection of established tumors. Cancer Research. 2016;**76**(8):2087-2093

[65] Daher M et al. CAR-NK cells: The next wave of cellular therapy for cancer. Clinical & Translational Immunology. 2021;**10**(4):e1274

[66] Yoon SR, Kim TD, Choi I. Understanding of molecular mechanisms in natural killer cell therapy. Experimental & Molecular Medicine. 2015;**47**(2):e141

[67] Damele L et al. Cord blood-derived natural killer cell exploitation in immunotherapy protocols: More than a promise? Cancers (Basel). 2022;**14**(18):4439

[68] Mehta RS, Shpall EJ, Rezvani K. Cord blood as a source of natural killer cells. Frontiers in Medicine (Lausanne). 2015;**2**:93

[69] Rafei H, Basar R, Acharya S, Zhang P, Liu P, Moseley SM, et al. Targeting T-cell lymphoma using CD70-directed cord blood-derived CAR-NK cells. Blood. 2023;**142**:4811

[70] Wilk AJ et al. Charge-altering releasable transporters enable phenotypic manipulation of natural killer cells for cancer immunotherapy. Blood Advances. 2020;**4**(17):4244-4255

[71] Liu S et al. NK cell-based cancer immunotherapy: From basic biology to clinical development. Journal of Hematology & Oncology. 2021;**14**(1):7

[72] Schmidt P, Raftery MJ, Pecher G. Engineering NK cells for CAR therapy-recent advances in gene transfer methodology. Frontiers in Immunology. 2020;**11**:611163

[73] Chang YH et al. A chimeric receptor with NKG2D specificity enhances natural killer cell activation and killing of tumor cells. Cancer Research. 2013;**73**(6):1777-1786

[74] Ng YY, Tay JCK, Wang S. CXCR1 expression to improve anti-cancer efficacy of intravenously injected CAR-NK cells in mice with peritoneal xenografts. Molecular Therapy - Oncolytics. 2020;**16**:75-85

[75] Xiao L et al. Adoptive transfer of NKG2D CAR mRNA-engineered

natural killer cells in colorectal cancer patients. Molecular Therapy. 2019;**27**(6):1114-1125

[76] Liu E et al. Use of CAR-transduced natural killer cells in CD19-positive lymphoid tumors. The New England Journal of Medicine. 2020;**382**(6):545-553

[77] M.D. Clinical trial information. Anderson Cancer Center; Available from: https://clinicaltrials.gov/study/NCT05092451

[78] Li L et al. Loss of metabolic fitness drives tumor resistance after CAR-NK cell therapy and can be overcome by cytokine engineering. Science Advances. 2023;**9**(30):eadd6997

[79] Li Y et al. KIR-based inhibitory CARs overcome CAR-NK cell trogocytosis-mediated fratricide and tumor escape. Nature Medicine. 2022;**28**(10):2133-2144

[80] Wculek SK et al. Dendritic cells in cancer immunology and immunotherapy. Nature Reviews. Immunology. 2020;**20**(1):7-24

[81] Santos PM, Butterfield LH. Dendritic cell-based cancer vaccines. Journal of Immunology. 2018;**200**(2):443-449

[82] Lin MJ et al. Cancer vaccines: The next immunotherapy frontier. Nature Cancer. 2022;**3**(8):911-926

[83] Fu C et al. Dendritic cell-based vaccines against cancer: Challenges, advances and future opportunities. Immunological Investigations. 2022;**51**(8):2133-2158

[84] Handy CE, Antonarakis ES. Sipuleucel-T for the treatment of prostate cancer: Novel insights and future directions. Future Oncology. 2018;**14**(10):907-917

[85] Tanyi JL et al. Personalized cancer vaccine effectively mobilizes antitumor T cell immunity in ovarian cancer. Science Translational Medicine. 2018;**10**(436):eaao5931

[86] Anguille S et al. Dendritic cell vaccination as postremission treatment to prevent or delay relapse in acute myeloid leukemia. Blood. 2017;**130**(15):1713-1721

[87] Wilgenhof S et al. Phase II study of autologous monocyte-derived mRNA electroporated dendritic cells (TriMixDC-MEL) plus ipilimumab in patients with pretreated advanced melanoma. Journal of Clinical Oncology. 2016;**34**(12):1330-1338

[88] Sundarasetty BS et al. Lentivirus-induced 'Smart' dendritic cells: Pharmacodynamics and GMP-compliant production for immunotherapy against TRP2-positive melanoma. Gene Therapy. 2015;**22**(9):707-720

[89] Han D et al. Anti-tumour immunity controlled through mRNA m(6)a methylation and YTHDF1 in dendritic cells. Nature. 2019;**566**(7743):270-274

[90] Lee JM et al. Phase I trial of intratumoral injection of CCL21 gene-modified dendritic cells in lung cancer elicits tumor-specific immune responses and CD8(+) T-cell infiltration. Clinical Cancer Research. 2017;**23**(16):4556-4568

[91] Pietrobon V et al. Improving CAR T-cell persistence. International Journal of Molecular Sciences. 2021;**22**(19):10828

[92] Chen GM et al. Integrative bulk and single-cell profiling of premanufacture T-cell populations reveals factors mediating long-term persistence of CAR T-cell therapy. Cancer Discovery. 2021;**11**(9):2186-2199

[93] Doan A et al. FOXO1 is a master regulator of CAR T memory programming. Research Square. 2023

[94] Tallantyre EC et al. Neurological updates: Neurological complications of CAR-T therapy. Journal of Neurology. 2021;**268**(4):1544-1554

[95] Flugel CL et al. Overcoming on-target, off-tumour toxicity of CAR T cell therapy for solid tumours. Nature Reviews. Clinical Oncology. 2023;**20**(1):49-62

[96] Andorko JI et al. Targeted in vivo generation of CAR T and NK Cells utilizing an engineered lentiviral vector platform. Blood. 2023;**142**:763

[97] Michels KR et al. Preclinical proof of concept for VivoVec, a lentiviral-based platform for in vivo CAR T-cell engineering. Journal for Immunotherapy of Cancer. 2023;**11**(3)

Chapter 3

Targeting Tumor Microenvironment for Advanced Cancer Therapy

Kuangyi Zhou, Tigran Sahakyan, Yuning Chen, Tyler Halladay, Niels Dawson, Sasha Semaan, Fujia Guo, Alba Mendis, Angela Song, Malianna Bahar Jazari, Truman Ma, Yan-Ruide Li and Lili Yang

Abstract

The tumor microenvironment (TME) has emerged as a pivotal determinant in the progression of cancer and the development of resistance to therapeutic interventions. The heterogeneous cellular composition of the TME not only facilitates tumor proliferation but also poses formidable obstacles to the efficacy of conventional treatments. This chapter delves into an examination of the distinctive attributes of the TME, exploring both established and innovative approaches designed to target the TME. Through a thorough analysis of the intricate involvement of the TME in cancer biology, we underscore the imperative for a comprehensive understanding and specific modulation of the TME to enhance the efficacy of cancer treatments. This elucidation provides novel insights for further research endeavors and clinical applications.

Keywords: tumor microenvironment (TME), cancer immunotherapy, tumor-associated macrophage (TAM), myeloid-derived suppressor cells (MDSC), cancer-associated fibroblasts (CAFs), extracellular matrix, therapy resistance, cancer progression, checkpoint blockade, chimeric antigen receptor (CAR)-engineered T (CAR-T) cell, innate T cell

1. Introduction

Contrary to the traditional view of cancer as a simple disease, cancer is now recognized as a complex ecosystem [1]. Besides cancer cells, the tumor microenvironment (TME), comprising a varied assortment of immune cells, cancer-associated fibroblasts (CAFs), endothelial cells (ECs), pericytes, and other cell types unique to tissue, plays a vital role in the development and treatment of cancer [2]. The cellular composition and functional condition of the TME may vary based on the tumor locations, the intrinsic traits of the cancer cells, the stage of the tumor, and patient-specific factors; within the TME, different cells could either inhibit or promote tumor

 IntechOpen

development [2]. Through heterotypic intercellular interactions between cancer and non-cancerous cells, TME diminishes the effectiveness of immune checkpoint blockade and adoptive cell therapies, underscoring the necessity of new treatments specifically designed to rectify the TME [3–5]. Given that TME contributes to the development and preservation of cancer hallmarks, including sustained proliferative signaling, resistance to cell death, angiogenesis induction, activation of invasion and metastasis, initiation of tumor-promoting inflammation, and evasion of immune destruction, to different extents, strategies targeting the TME have become a significant focus in antitumor therapy, which includes targeting tumor-infiltrating T-cells, confronting cancer-associated fibroblasts, modulating the extracellular matrix, and so on [6–9].

This chapter offers a thorough introduction to the major composition and corresponding dynamic interactions within the TME, which subsequently affects cancer progression and antitumor therapy resistance. Current techniques targeting the TME along with their effectiveness and clinical applications are discussed. Moreover, this chapter explores innovative approaches in advanced cancer therapy that incorporate TME considerations. Finally, this chapter evaluates the synergistic effects of combining TME targeting with conventional cancer treatments, providing a comprehensive overview of the strategies to improve cancer therapy through TME modulation.

2. Key components in the TME

Cancerous cells are not the only ones involved in the development and progression of the disease [1]. In fact, the TME is made up of a wide variety of cell types and other components that function to both support and resist cancer progression [4, 6, 10, 11]. Of these components, the most important ones include immune cells, stromal cells, vascular cells, as well as the extracellular matrix [2]. It is the interaction between these cells and tumor cells that make the TME a rich ecosystem for cancer development and resistance against the immune system [12]. The section below outlines the key elements that comprise the TME and highlights how they function in the scope of tumorigenesis.

Among the most diverse subset of cells in the TME are cells of the innate and adaptive immune systems [3]. The innate immune cells—macrophages, neutrophils, invariant natural killer T cells—present the body's first line of defense and utilize non-specific mechanisms to fight pathogens, including cancer [13]. On the other hand, adaptive immune cells, such as B cells, T cells, and natural killer cells, are highly specific in their targeting of pathogens [13]. While some of these cells possess potent antitumor properties, such as the highly cytotoxic natural killer cells and CD8-positive T cells, others like the immunosuppressive regulatory T cells and M2-like macrophages actually support the growth of the tumor by preventing inflammation and participating in the formation of new blood vessels [2].

Adding to the complexity of the constantly evolving TME are stromal cells and vascular cells [8, 14, 15]. Typically, stromal cells are found surrounding organs and act as structural tissue to protect and support them [14]. Depending on their origin, stromal cells can be identified as cancer associated fibroblasts, adipocytes, and stellate cells [13]. In the context of tumorigenesis, cancer cells recruit the stromal cells of their surrounding tissue and incorporate the plasticity and regulatory signaling of these cells to the advantage of the tumor [14]. For example, cancer-associated fibroblasts are a major component of the TME that exhibit enhanced proliferative and extracellular matrix formation upon activation [14]. They can be formed from a variety of stromal cells, including adipocytes and stellate cells of the liver, as well as mesenchymal stem cells derived from the bone marrow [13]. Due to their ability to model the extracellular matrix, cancer-associated fibroblasts can influence the mode of interaction among the subtypes of cells in the TME and directly change the mechanical properties of the tumor as a whole [13, 16]. Additionally, stromal cells contribute to the growth of cancer through the secretion of pro-inflammatory cytokines and growth factors for the promotion of blood vessel formation [14]. Since most solid tumors tend to develop hypoxic conditions, blood vessel formation, also known as angiogenesis, is essential for the progression of cancer [2]. Therefore, it is not surprising that vascular cells such as endothelial cells contribute largely to the TME. In an otherwise nutrient-deprived setting, tumors utilize vascular endothelial cells to form new blood vessels that can deliver them essential nourishment [13].

Apart from the multiple cell types present in the TME, an important factor of the ecosystem is the extracellular matrix [14]. Comprised of proteins, glycoproteins, and collagen, the extracellular matrix not only provides structure to the TME but also forms the space in which cancer cells interact with all the other cell types [2]. This includes facilitating contact-dependent communication between cells and acting as a reservoir for secreted cytokines and signaling molecules to be detected by cells in the vicinity [2]. For example, in the latter case, the extracellular matrix may sequester growth factors such as vascular endothelial growth factor (VEGF) that promotes angiogenesis, which can bind to endothelial cells and initiate blood vessel formation in the tumor [13].

The TME is a highly dynamic phenomenon, with all of the components—cellular or molecular—functioning together for the cancer to survive and grow [17]. Cancer cells recruit their surrounding cells to develop defenses and to utilize the host system for their benefit [17]. Immune cells are polarized to become immunosuppressive, as is the case of M2-like macrophages [17]. These macrophages promote angiogenesis in the tumor through the secretion of the VEGF and suppress antitumor immune cells such as T helper cells by secreting anti-inflammatory cytokines like IL-10 [12]. In addition to interactions between cancer cells and the other cells of the TME, the interplay between the non-tumor components is another crucial factor that drives the tumor progression as well as resistance [14]. As stromal cells can be transformed into proliferative cancer-associated fibroblasts, which in turn drive the formation of the tumor extracellular matrix, they also signal to vascular endothelial cells to form new blood vessels [12]. On another level, the same cancer-associated fibroblasts involved in the structural formation of the tumor also suppress cytotoxic T cells through the secretion of the anti-inflammatory cytokine TGF-β [18]. This way, the cancer delegates its own development to the cells of the TME and utilizes intrinsic mechanisms found in them to confer resistance against the antitumor immune response and therapies in development [12].

Currently, there is a lack of treatments targeting the TME in standard clinical use [13]. The TME then arises as a critical barrier to effective treatment, due to the TME milieu being central to several pathways responsible for drug resistance, tumor metastasis, growth, and immune evasion [17]. Therefore, surmounting the obstacles posed by the TME presents a promising therapeutic strategy that could substantially enhance the success of solid tumor therapies [13]. Outlined below are the various therapy strategies that concurrently target the TME and tumors and demonstrate synergistic effects with enhanced efficacy (**Figure 1**).

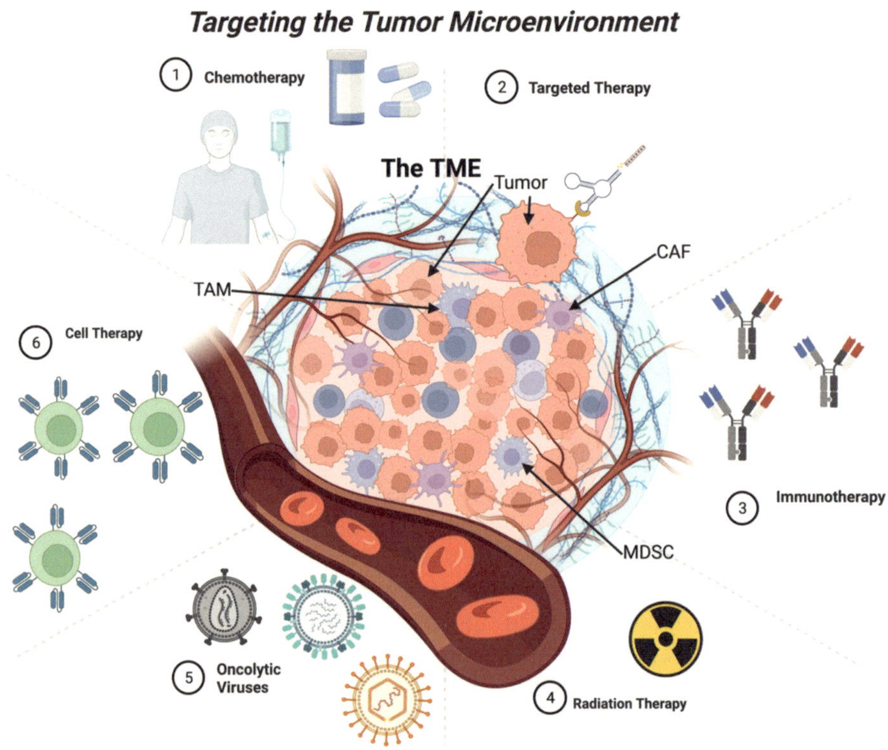

Figure 1.
Multiple strategies to target the tumor microenvironment.

3. Chemotherapy, targeted therapy, and immunotherapy to target the TME

Cytotoxic agents such as Taxols, cisplatin, and 5-fluorouracil are the cornerstones of cancer therapy due to their ability to disrupt essential physiological processes such as cell division, metabolic processes, and DNA replication in rapidly proliferating cells [19]. Despite their demonstrated effectiveness, chemotherapies face a significant hurdle in the form of the TME, which limits their cytotoxic potential [17]. Thus, most current strategies employed to minimize the effects of the TME combine chemotherapy, targeted therapy, and immunotherapy, specifically targeting immunosuppressive components within the TME to enhance the overall efficacy of cancer treatments [17].

3.1 Depletion of TAMs

Tumor-associated macrophages (TAMs) exhibit the capability to rescue and promote the survival of cancer cells post-exposure to antimitotic agents, such as Taxols, which disrupt microtubule dynamics crucial for successful cell division [20]. By curtailing the duration of Taxol-induced mitotic arrest and mitigating the activation of apoptosis pathways prompted by Taxols, TAMs play a pivotal role in preventing cancer cell death *via* the secretion of specific factors [20]. Therefore, blocking the CSF-1/CSF1R axis to prevent M2-like polarization and TAM recruitment emerges as a strategy to counteract the effects of TAMs [21]. Investigations of breast cancer focusing on depleting TAMs within the TME through CSF-1R inhibition have demonstrated increased DNA damage and amplified cancer cell death when combined with Taxol treatment compared to Taxol treatment alone [20].

The blocking of PD-1/PD-L1 with monoclonal antibodies is well established as a potent therapy for a diversity of cancers [22–26]. TAM expression of PD-1 in the TME has been shown to inhibit macrophage phagocytosis and tumor immunity [27]. However, TAM infiltration is also associated with PD-1/PD-L1 checkpoint inhibitor (CI) immunotherapy drug resistance by secreting immunosuppressive cytokines and metabolic products and increasing the surface expression of PD-L1 on tumor cells [28, 29]. Given these caveats in the context of TAM activity in PD-1/PD-L1 therapy, combination therapy targeting TAM depletion offers an innovative alternative. In fact, using both CSF-1R inhibitors and PD-L1/PD-1 CI immunotherapy has shown promise in treating brain cancers [28, 30, 31]. Likewise, clinical trials implementing a combined regimen of chemotherapy and antibodies that obstruct signals involved in TAM recruitment, such as CCR2, have observed synergistic effects [32]. Another immunotherapy currently in several clinical trials includes a CD40 agonist, also known as mitazalimab, which aims to reprogram TAMs toward an antitumor M1-like state and away from an M2-like immunosuppressive state, thereby increasing penetration of cytotoxic T cells and chemotherapeutic agents into the tumor stroma [33, 34]. Finally, V domain Ig suppressor of T cell activation (VISTA), an Ig superfamily protein primarily found in the hematopoietic compartment, has been investigated for its involvement in negatively regulating T cell responses [35, 36]. VISTA knockout on macrophages and myeloid-derived suppressor cells (MDSCs) resulted in a reduced ability to locate to the TME [37]. VISTA CI immunotherapy has shown promise alone and in conjunction with PD-1/PD-L1 CI immunotherapy [38]. These studies underscore the active role the TME plays in facilitating tumor progression and survival and emphasize the need to target both the TME and tumor.

3.2 Depletion of MDSCs

MDSCs are a heterogeneous population of immature myeloid cells known to rapidly proliferate in the TME [39]. MDSCs are further defined into two subsets based on their phenotype, morphology, and activity: polymorphonuclear (PMN)-MDSCs and monocytic (M)-MDSCs [39, 40]. The proliferation of MDSCs is driven by tumor-derived growth factors, including GM-CSF, G-CSF, M-CSF, VEGF, and IL-6 [41]. The most notable and unique characteristic of MDSCs is their plasticity [42]. MDSCs can act on many cell types at once, including by differentiating into TAMs, suppressive DCs, and M2-like suppressive macrophages [42]. Strategies for targeting MDSCs include depletion by chemotherapy and CD33-targeted antibody-drug conjugate therapy, differentiation by TLR agonists such as CpG oligonucleotides, blocking accumulation by chemokine inhibitors and STAT3 inhibitors, and directly blocking immunosuppression through PDE5 inhibitors and COX2 inhibitors [42]. Moreover, combinations of several of these therapies can provide new effective therapies for testing in clinical trials. One such clinical trial involves the use of a TLR agonist known as MGN1703 in conjunction with a CTLA-4 monoclonal antibody in late-stage solid tumor malignancies [43]. Another study sought to treat metastatic triple-negative breast cancer by delivering a combinational therapy of a TLR3 ligand called rintatolimod, IFN-a2b, and a COX-2 inhibitor called celecoxib, which resulted in a significant increase in cytotoxic T lymphocyte infiltration into the TME and clinical and stable disease responses in patients [44]. As more clinical trials are undertaken, one case study highlights the unique promise offered by combination therapies. A patient who had experienced hepatic metastases of metastatic sinonasal undifferentiated carcinoma progression following treatment with pembrolizumab (PD-1 inhibitor) was treated with an additional combined regimen of ipilimumab (CTLA-4 inhibitor) and COX-2 inhibitor, resulting in a clinical response in target liver metastases [45].

3.3 Modulation of regulatory T cells

Regulatory T cells are the primary T cells (Tregs) responsible for immunosuppression in the TME [46]. They have been identified as major obstacles to the immune response in the TME because they secrete inhibitory cytokines and directly inhibit antitumor immune cells such as cytotoxic $CD8^{+}$ T lymphocytes [46]. The most common immunotherapy targeting tumor-infiltrating lymphocytes (TILs) is immune checkpoint inhibitors (ICIs) (CTLA-4, TIGIT, and PD-1), which have achieved success [47]. Notably, 60-70% of patients receiving PD-1 ICI therapy do not experience an objective response, with 20-30% of patients experiencing eventual tumor relapse [47–50]. At the same time, depletion of Tregs is associated with a number of autoimmune diseases [51]. Thus, some scientists have called for a combination therapy of Treg depletion by CD25 and CCR8 and ICI therapy to improve outcome and prevent complete organism-wide depletion of Tregs [50]. In addition to these therapies, the development of the GITR agonist is of note. GITR has been identified as a possible co-stimulator on Tregs and is highly expressed on the surface of Tregs [50, 52]. When stimulated by its ligand, DTA-1, Tregs become apoptotic [50, 52]. Recent clinical trials have shown anti-GITR products are not effective in reducing cancer burdens, but new PD-1, anti-GITR multimers have shown promise in *in vivo* mouse models [50, 52].

3.4 Blocking of dysfunctional angiogenesis

Abnormal angiogenesis fosters a vascular network designed to bolster tumor development, metastasis, and the sustenance of the tumor *via* nutrient supply [53]. Among the major drivers of this process lies the vascular endothelial growth factor (VEGF) pathway [53]. Tumor cells commonly overexpress VEGF and engage this pathway as VEGF binds to its respective receptor on endothelial cells, thereby stimulating their proliferation and formation of erratic blood vessels [54]. The aberrant vasculature within tumors diminishes the effects of chemotherapeutic drugs *via* two modalities: 1. Reduction of cellular apoptosis and 2. Impairment of drug delivery into tumor sites [54]. Consequently, blocking the VEGF pathway offers a strategy to potentiate the efficacy of chemotherapeutic drugs [54]. Notably, in a phase III trial for colorectal cancer, combining antibodies against VEGF, like bevacizumab, with chemotherapy (irinotecan, 5-FU, and leucovorin), yielded significantly improved overall survival and progression-free survival compared to treatments without bevacizumab [54]. Multiple clinical trials for other indications including breast cancer and non-small cell lung cancer have also replicated these similar synergistic effects and overall highlight the impact of concurrently targeting the TME alongside the tumor itself [54].

3.5 Targeting hypoxia and metabolites

A hypoxic TME is an intrinsic characteristic of solid malignant tumors. As cancer cells proliferate, they rapidly consume oxygen [55]. Moreover, abnormal vasculature further contributes to a hypoxic environment, increasing the likelihood of metastasis, resistance to traditional cancer therapies, and a poor prognosis [42]. Tumor cells can survive in such an environment by switching to anerobic metabolism, producing erythropoietin, and upregulating proto-oncogenes [56]. Additionally, hypoxia has been shown to contribute to the function and accumulation of intra-tumoral Tregs and tumor-associated macrophages, further suppressing the immune response [57]. Specifically, unlike activated effector T cells, Tregs primarily rely on oxidative phosphorylation and fatty acid oxidation, metabolic processes favored by the hypoxic, low pH, and nutrient-depleted TME [58]. Cancer immunotherapies target this difference in metabolism using checkpoint blockades (CTLA-4, PD-1) and lactate neutralizers (MCT inhibitors or pH-selective antibodies) [58]. Numerous hypoxia-inducible factor targeting drugs interfere with hypoxia-inducible factors during various stages of their production [16, 59]. Some approaches include inhibiting HIF-1α mRNA expression, preventing HIF-1α translation, degrading HIF-1α protein, and interfering with HIF-1α and HIF-2α heterodimerization with HIF-1β to impair hypoxic tumor growth [60]. Another therapy exploits the hypoxic environment to deliver cytotoxins. Hypoxia-activated prodrugs are reduced by cellular oxidoreductases to form DNA-reactive cytotoxins through a process irreversible only in hypoxic conditions [61, 62]. These DNA-reactive cytotoxins then proceed to kill hypoxic cancer cells [16, 59]. Although some hypoxia-activated prodrugs showed promise in Phase I and II clinical trials, there has been limited success in Phase III trials. TH-302, a prodrug that releases isophosphoramide mustard, which alkylates DNA under hypoxia, has shown considerable promise among hypoxia-activated prodrugs and is under combinational therapy clinical trials [61]. Furthermore, hyperoxia therapy aims to increase oxygen content to reverse tumor hypoxia through various methods, including hyperbaric oxygen therapy, normobaric oxygen therapy, carbogen inhalation, and oxygen-generating nanoparticles, among others [16, 59]. Supplementing oxygen to reduce hypoxia is still in its nascent stages of investigation and is being explored for combinational therapies [59].

4. Radiation therapy to target the TME

The use of high doses of radiation to irreparably damage the DNA of cancer cells is a common therapy that approximately 50% of all cancer patients receive and contribute toward 40% of cured cancers [63]. However, the benefits of radiation therapy are offset by the concomitant remodeling of the TME into a more immunosuppressive one, as exemplified by the indirect boost of tumor-promoting TAM infiltration during radiation [64]. One promising way to address this challenge is by combining radiation therapy with TME-specific treatments. For instance, blocking immunosuppressive pathways during radiation can significantly enhance antitumor activity while attenuating radiotherapy side effects such as tissue scarring [65]. Additionally, tumor cells can be further sensitized to irradiation through the use of nanoparticles [66]. Manganese dioxide (MnO2) has been shown to increase the pH of the TME and reduce hypoxic conditions, thus inhibiting tumor autophagy [66, 67]. Indeed, subsequent *in vivo* studies combining MnO2 nanoparticles with radiation therapy demonstrated a significant decrease in tumor growth compared to radiation alone [66]. These recent developments in radiation therapy illustrate how combining it with TME-specific treatments could greatly improve tumor-eradicating efficacy while diminishing radiation's undesired side effects.

5. Oncolytic viruses to target the TME

The effectiveness of oncolytic viruses (OVs) relies on their ability to selectively target tumor cells. For instance, HSV-based oncolytics such as T-VEC (Imlygic) and Delytact achieve tumor specificity through the deletion of specific genes to prevent antiviral pathways and inhibit virus-mediated inhibition, proving clinically successful [68]. Another example is Vaccinia virus (VV)-based oncolytics, exemplified by JX594 and derivatives, which have shown varying degrees of efficacy in late-phase clinical trials [69, 70]. Their natural tropism toward tumor cells, coupled with genetic modifications such as thymidine kinase (TK) gene deletion, enhances tumor selectivity [68]. OVs play a crucial role in transforming the immunologically cold TME into an immunologically hot environment [71]. This shift promotes long-term tumor-specific immunity, providing surveillance against relapse [71]. OV therapy influences the dendritic cell-T cell axis by inducing immunogenic cell death, releasing damage-associated molecular patterns (DAMPs), pathogen-associated molecular patterns (PAMPs), and cytokines [72]. Dendritic cells (DCs) are potent antigen-presenting cells that bridge the innate and adaptive immune systems [73]. OV therapy enhances DC infiltration, maturation, and antigen presentation, promoting T cell activation [74]. CAFs within the TME impede the spread of viruses within the ECM, limiting the effectiveness of oncolytic viruses alone [75]. To address this challenge, an oncolytic adenovirus with a modified gene (Rb-binding-deleted E1A), controlled by a promoter derived from the stroma-related SPARC gene, successfully infected and destroyed both tumor and stromal cells in experiments involving human ovarian cancer and stroma-containing tumors in mice, without causing harm to non-malignant tissues [75]. In addition to CAFs, immunosuppressive cells in the TME, such as Tregs and TAMs, can limit the efficacy of oncolytic viruses [76]. Scientists are addressing this challenge by targeting these cells using oncolytic viruses engineered to express immunomodulatory agents [76]. An illustrative study identified Folate Receptor B (FRb) as a marker on M2-like macrophages *in vitro* [76]. FRb-targeted oncolytic viruses demonstrated the ability to activate the body's own T cells and reduce the number of M2-like macrophages in samples taken from cancer patients with malignant ascites, thus preserving the more pro-inflammatory M1-like macrophages [77]. The combination of tumor-selective replication and immunomodulation by oncolytic viruses offers a flexible approach to combating cancer [78]. Their combination to overcome the TME shows promise, underscoring the changing field of oncolytic viral therapy for more potent cancer treatments.

6. Cell-based therapies to target the TME

The use of chimeric antigen receptor (CAR)-engineered T (CAR-T) cell therapy has emerged as a groundbreaking approach to treat blood cancers and is now rising as a potential therapy for solid tumors [11, 79]. The therapy entails the extraction of T cells from cancer patients, subsequent enhancement of these T cells through the induction of CAR molecules, and the autologous re-infusion of the enhanced T cells [11, 79]. Despite demonstrating substantial promise in addressing solid tumors, akin to numerous therapies, cell-based therapies are met with challenges posed by the TME. Major obstacles inhibiting the efficacy of cell-based therapies include the immunosuppressive nature and hindered infiltration of the TME [3, 17, 80, 81]. Physical barriers within the TME, such as TAMs, ECM, and irregular vasculature, restrict the ability of cell-based therapies to infiltrate this milieu [3, 17, 80, 81]. Moreover, a multitude of immunosuppressive elements, including immunosuppressive cells such as TAMs, MDSCs, and Tregs, alongside inhibitory molecules such as PD-L1, CTLA-4, adenosine, TGFB, and IL-10, among others, are ubiquitous within the TME [82]. These immunosuppressive components facilitate T cell exhaustion and dampen the immune response [5]. Innovative strategies have emerged to disrupt the TME, representing the next generation of cell products designed to treat solid tumors.

6.1 TAM targeting innate-like T cells

TAMs constitute a substantial portion of the TME, often comprising up to 50% of the tumor mass in some tumors [13]. These TAMs play a dual role: 1. Act as a physical barrier that hinders immune cell infiltration and 2. Express high levels of PD-L1, inducing T cell exhaustion, contributing significantly to maintaining an immunosuppressive TME [3, 17]. Traditional CAR-T cell therapy relies on conventional αβ T cells sourced from cancer patients due to their intrinsic cytotoxic properties [83]. However, these T cells pose the risk of graft versus host disease (GvHD) and lack the capacity to remodel the TME [84]. To address these limitations, an innovative strategy involves leveraging unconventional T cells equipped with CARs. These unconventional T cells, including invariant natural killer (iNKT), mucosal-associated invariant T (MAIT), and gamma-delta T (γδT) cells, are MHC-I independent and possess TCRs that recognize distinct antigen-presenting molecules CD1d, MR1, and BTN3A1 (CD277), respectively [3–5]. Importantly, these antigen-presenting molecules are highly conserved and ubiquitously expressed on TAMs [5]. Unconventional T cells engage in a TCR-dependent mechanism that enables them to target and eliminate TAMs effectively, remodeling the TME toward a more proinflammatory state [3–5]. Through engineering with CARs, these unconventional T cells can simultaneously modulate the TME and target the tumor itself, potentially enhancing the efficacy of solid tumor therapies [5].

6.2 MDSC targeting CAR-T cells

Another challenge to CAR-T therapy lies in MDSCs, a heterogeneous immune cell population recruited to the TME of most solid tumors [3–5]. MDSCs inhibit effector T cell activity through multiple mechanisms, such as promoting Treg expansion, secreting immunosuppressive cytokines, and sequestering essential amino acids for T cell proliferation [3–5]. One approach to rescue CAR-T cytotoxicity could be in the engineering of a chimeric receptor targeting both MDSCs and tumor cells. As agonists of TRAIL Receptor 2 (TR2) selectively induce apoptosis in MDSCs, engineering CAR-T cells with TR2 is a promising strategy [85]. *In vitro* studies demonstrated that adding TR2 and co-stimulatory receptor 41BB on CAR-T cells decreased the numbers of MDSCs while significantly enhancing CAR-T cell potency against tumor cells [85]. In comparison, CAR-T cells targeting either MDSCs or tumor cells alone did not prove as effective [85]. This synergistic approach to CAR-T cell engineering emphasizes the benefits of simultaneously targeting cancer cells and their microenvironment.

6.3 ECM degrading CAR-T cells

Cell-based therapies targeting tumor cells are limited by the extent of their infiltration into the TME [5]. The ECM plays a major role in shaping the TME, influencing its histopathology, behavior, and governing biochemical and biophysical aspects regulating TME processes [5]. Besides facilitating cancer progression and metastasis, the ECM acts as a physical barrier impeding immune cell infiltration, thereby diminishing the effectiveness of various cell-based therapies [86]. To address this obstacle, innovative engineering approaches have emerged to overexpress heparanase (HPSE), an enzyme that degrades heparan sulfate proteoglycans (HSPGs), a key ECM constituent [86]. Disrupting the ECM *via* HPSE overexpression promotes immune cell infiltration [86]. This modification, incorporated alongside CAR engineering in T cells, demonstrated enhanced infiltration and antitumor efficacy in preclinical xenograft models of neuroblastoma for GD2-specific CAR-T cells with HPSE engineering [86]. This engineering approach highlights the significance of concurrently targeting the TME and tumor cells, perpetuating synergistic effects overcoming TME limitations.

6.4 Blocking immunosuppressive molecules with ICB

In the TME, cell-based therapies encounter challenges from immunosuppressive molecules inducing cellular exhaustion and diminished cytotoxicity, reducing the effectiveness of therapies for solid tumors [5]. Among these molecules, PD-L1 stands out as a prominent checkpoint ligand ubiquitously expressed within the TME by macrophages, DCs, MDSCs, B and T cells, fibroblasts, and tumor cells [87, 88]. The binding of PD-L1 with PD1 expressed on therapeutic cells deactivates the immune response and cellular activation by inhibiting proliferation, inducing cell death, diminishing persistence, and decreasing effector function [23, 88, 89]. Blocking the immunosuppressive interaction between PD-1 of immune cells and PD-L1 within the TME offers synergistic effects with cell-based therapies against solid tumors [4]. Preclinical models of $Her2^{+}$ sarcoma and breast cancer demonstrated synergistic effects where combining anti-PD-1 and Her2-targeting T cells resulted in enhanced CAR-T cell function and tumor killing [87]. The combination of immune checkpoint blockade and CAR-T cell therapy synergizes by blocking the immunosuppressive PD-1 axis between the therapeutic cells and TME, improving therapeutic outcomes compared to CAR-T cell therapy alone [4].

7. Conclusion

In this chapter, we conduct a thorough examination of the TME in the progression and treatment of cancer. Far from being a bystander, the TME is characterized by its complex and dynamic interactions, actively participating in the context of cancer. TME exerts a significant influence on tumor development, metastasis, and the efficacy of therapeutic interventions. The intricate relationship between the TME and cancer cells introduces distinct challenges while also unveiling new opportunities for enhancing cancer treatment strategies.

Despite the variety, numerous cancer therapies such as radiation, chemotherapy, and cell-based treatments are commonly limited by the TME. By significantly contributing to cancer growth and survival, the TME often reduces the efficacy of cancer-targeting therapies. Strategies that simultaneously address both cancer cells themselves and the TME have shown promise in effectively treating solid tumors. The development of innovative methods to target the TME offers the potential for enhancing cancer treatments. Such advancements could enhance patient outcomes and overcome the challenges presented by the TME in cancer therapy.

Overall, this chapter highlights the critical role of TME in cancer. Integrating a comprehensive understanding of the TME is necessary for the development of cancer treatment strategies. The multifaceted consideration offers insights for further research and clinical applications that could bolster the efficacy of cancer therapies.

Acknowledgements

We thank the lab members from Dr. Lili Yang's lab (UCLA) for their insightful discussion.

Authors' contributions

K.Z., T.S., and Y.C. wrote the manuscript with the assistance of T.H., N.D., S.S., F.G., A.M., A.S., M.B.J., T.M. Y.-R.L. and L.Y. reviewed and edited the manuscript.

Funding

This work was supported by a UCLA BSCRC Innovation Award (to L.Y.) and an Ablon Scholars Award (to L.Y.). Y.-R.L. was a postdoctoral fellow supported by a UCLA MIMG M. John Pickett Post-Doctoral Fellow Award and a CIRM-BSCRC Postdoctoral Fellowship.

Competing interests

L.Y. is a scientific advisor to AlzChem and Amberstone Biosciences and a co-founder, stockholder, and advisory board member of Appia Bio. None of the declared companies contributed to or directed any of the writing of this manuscript. The authors declare no competing interests.

Author details

Kuangyi Zhou[1†], Tigran Sahakyan[1†], Yuning Chen[1†], Tyler Halladay[1], Niels Dawson[1], Sasha Semaan[1], Fujia Guo[1], Alba Mendis[1], Angela Song[1], Malianna Bahar Jazari[1], Truman Ma[1], Yan-Ruide Li[1*] and Lili Yang[1,2,3,4*]

1 Department of Microbiology, Immunology and Molecular Genetics, University of California, Los Angeles, CA, USA

2 Eli and Edythe Broad Center of Regenerative Medicine and Stem Cell Research, University of California, Los Angeles, CA, USA

3 Jonsson Comprehensive Cancer Center, David Geffen School of Medicine, University of California, Los Angeles, CA, USA

4 Molecular Biology Institute, University of California, Los Angeles, CA, USA

*Address all correspondence to: charlie.li@ucla.edu and liliyang@ucla.edu

† These authors contributed equally.

References

[1] Chen X, Song E. The theory of tumor ecosystem. Cancer Communications (London, England). 2022;**42**:587-608

[2] de Visser KE, Joyce JA. The evolving tumor microenvironment: From cancer initiation to metastatic outgrowth. Cancer Cell. 2023;**41**:374-403

[3] Li Y-R, Wilson M, Yang L. Target tumor microenvironment by innate T cells. Frontiers in Immunology. 2022;**13**:999549

[4] Li Y-R, Yu Y, Kramer A, Hon R, Wilson M, Brown J, et al. An ex vivo 3D tumor microenvironment-mimicry culture to study TAM modulation of cancer immunotherapy. Cell. 2022;**11**:1583

[5] Li Y-R, Brown J, Yu Y, Lee D, Zhou K, Dunn ZS, et al. Targeting immunosuppressive tumor-associated macrophages using innate T cells for enhanced antitumor reactivity. Cancers. 2022;**14**:2749

[6] Li Y-R, Fang Y, Lyu Z, Zhu Y, Yang L. Exploring the dynamic interplay between cancer stem cells and the tumor microenvironment: Implications for novel therapeutic strategies. Journal of Translational Medicine. 2023;**21**:686

[7] Pan Y, Yu Y, Wang X, Zhang T. Tumor-associated macrophages in tumor immunity. Frontiers in Immunology [Internet]. 2020. DOI: 10.3389/fimmu.2020.583084

[8] Choi J, Gyamfi J, Jang H, Koo JS. The role of tumor-associated macrophage in breast cancer biology. Histology and Histopathology. 2018;**33**:133-145

[9] Xiao Y, Yu D. Tumor microenvironment as a therapeutic target in cancer. Pharmacology & Therapeutics. 2021;**221**:107753

[10] Petitprez F, Meylan M, de Reyniès A, Sautès-Fridman C, Fridman WH. The tumor microenvironment in the response to immune checkpoint blockade therapies. Frontiers in Immunology. 2020;**11**:784

[11] Li Y-R, Ochoa CJ, Zhu Y, Kramer A, Wilson M, Fang Y, et al. Profiling ovarian cancer tumor and microenvironment during disease progression for cell-based immunotherapy design. iScience. 2023;**26**:107952

[12] Son B, Lee S, Youn H, Kim E, Kim W, Youn B. The role of tumor microenvironment in therapeutic resistance. Oncotarget. 2017;**8**:3933-3945

[13] Anderson NM, Simon MC. The tumor microenvironment. Current Biology. 2020;**30**:R921-R925

[14] Kalluri R. The biology and function of fibroblasts in cancer. Nature Reviews. Cancer. 2016;**16**:582-598

[15] Ribatti D. The involvement of endothelial progenitor cells in tumor angiogenesis. Journal of Cellular and Molecular Medicine. 2004;**8**:294-300

[16] Cirri P, Chiarugi P. Cancer-associated-fibroblasts and tumour cells: A diabolic liaison driving cancer progression. Cancer Metastasis Reviews. 2012;**31**:195-208

[17] Bejarano L, Jordão MJC, Joyce JA. Therapeutic targeting of the tumor microenvironment. Cancer Discovery. 2021;**11**:933-959

[18] Rouzbahani E, Majidpoor J, Najafi S, Mortezaee K. Cancer stem cells in immunoregulation and bypassing anti-checkpoint therapy. Biomedicine & Pharmacotherapy. 2022;**156**:113906

[19] Schirrmacher V. From chemotherapy to biological therapy: A review of novel concepts to reduce the side effects of systemic cancer treatment (review). International Journal of Oncology. 2019;**54**:407-419

[20] Olson OC, Kim H, Quail DF, Foley EA, Joyce JA. Tumor-associated macrophages suppress the cytotoxic activity of antimitotic agents. Cell Reports. 2017;**19**:101-113

[21] Ries CH, Cannarile MA, Hoves S, Benz J, Wartha K, Runza V, et al. Targeting tumor-associated macrophages with anti-CSF-1R antibody reveals a strategy for cancer therapy. Cancer Cell. 2014;**25**:846-859

[22] Zou W, Wolchok JD, Chen L. PD-L1 (B7-H1) and PD-1 pathway blockade for cancer therapy: Mechanisms, response biomarkers, and combinations. Science Translational Medicine. 2016;**8**:328rv4

[23] Pardoll DM. The blockade of immune checkpoints in cancer immunotherapy. Nature Reviews. Cancer. 2012;**12**:252-264

[24] Topalian SL, Hodi FS, Brahmer JR, Gettinger SN, Smith DC, McDermott DF, et al. Safety, activity, and immune correlates of anti-PD-1 antibody in cancer. The New England Journal of Medicine. 2012;**366**:2443-2454

[25] Topalian SL, Sznol M, McDermott DF, Kluger HM, Carvajal RD, Sharfman WH, et al. Survival, durable tumor remission, and long-term safety in patients with advanced melanoma receiving Nivolumab. Journal of Clinical Oncology: Official Journal of the American Society of Clinical Oncology. 2023;**41**:943-954

[26] Hamid O, Robert C, Daud A, Hodi FS, Hwu W-J, Kefford R, et al. Safety and tumor responses with lambrolizumab (anti-PD-1) in melanoma. The New England Journal of Medicine. 2013;**369**:134-144

[27] Gordon SR, Maute RL, Dulken BW, Hutter G, George BM, McCracken MN, et al. PD-1 expression by tumour-associated macrophages inhibits phagocytosis and tumour immunity. Nature. 2017;**545**:495-499

[28] Cui X, Ma C, Vasudevaraja V, Serrano J, Tong J, Peng Y, et al. Dissecting the immunosuppressive tumor microenvironments in glioblastoma-on-a-Chip for optimized PD-1 immunotherapy. eLife. 2020;**9**:e52253

[29] Pu Y, Ji Q. Tumor-associated macrophages regulate PD-1/PD-L1 immunosuppression. Frontiers in Immunology. 2022;**13**:874589

[30] Mao Y, Eissler N, Le BK, Johnsen JI, Kogner P, Kiessling R. Targeting suppressive myeloid cells potentiates checkpoint inhibitors to control spontaneous Neuroblastoma. Clinical Cancer Research: An Official Journal of the American Association for Cancer Research. 2016;**22**:3849-3859

[31] Liu Y, Zhan Z, Kang Z, Li M, Lv Y, Li S, et al. Preclinical and early clinical studies of a novel compound SYHA1813 that efficiently crosses the blood-brain barrier and exhibits potent activity against glioblastoma. Acta Pharmaceutica Sinica B. 2023;**13**:4748-4764

[32] Nywening TM, Wang-Gillam A, Sanford DE, Belt BA, Panni RZ, Cusworth BM, et al. Targeting tumour-associated macrophages with

CCR2 inhibition in combination with FOLFIRINOX in patients with borderline resectable and locally advanced pancreatic cancer: A single-Centre, open-label, dose-finding, non-randomised, phase 1b trial. The Lancet Oncology. 2016;**17**:651-662

[33] Cassetta L, Pollard JW. Targeting macrophages: Therapeutic approaches in cancer. Nature Reviews. Drug Discovery. 2018;**17**:887-904

[34] Prenen H, Borbath I, Geboes KP, Cassier PA, Lambert A, Mitry E, et al. Efficacy and safety of mitazalimab in combination with mFOLFIRINOX in patients with metastatic pancreatic ductal adenocarcinoma (mPDAC): An interim analysis of the optimize-1 phase 1b/2 study. Journal of Clinical Oncology [Internet]. 2023;**41**:4139. DOI: 10.1200/JCO.2023.41.16_suppl.4139

[35] Lines JL, Pantazi E, Mak J, Sempere LF, Wang L, O'Connell S, et al. VISTA is an immune checkpoint molecule for human T cells. Cancer Research. 2014;**74**:1924-1932

[36] Mehta N, Maddineni S, Mathews II, Andres Parra Sperberg R, Huang P-S, Cochran JR. Structure and functional binding epitope of V-domain Ig suppressor of T cell activation. Cell Reports. 2019;**28**:2509-2516.e5

[37] Broughton TWK, ElTanbouly MA, Schaafsma E, Deng J, Sarde A, Croteau W, et al. Defining the signature of VISTA on myeloid cell chemokine responsiveness. Frontiers in Immunology. 2019;**10**:2641

[38] Iadonato S, Ovechkina Y, Lustig K, Cross J, Eyde N, Frazier E, et al. A highly potent anti-VISTA antibody KVA12123 - A new immune checkpoint inhibitor and a promising therapy against poorly immunogenic tumors. Frontiers in Immunology. 2023;**14**:1311658

[39] Li K, Shi H, Zhang B, Ou X, Ma Q, Chen Y, et al. Myeloid-derived suppressor cells as immunosuppressive regulators and therapeutic targets in cancer. Signal Transduction and Targeted Therapy. 2021;**6**:362

[40] Bronte V, Brandau S, Chen S-H, Colombo MP, Frey AB, Greten TF, et al. Recommendations for myeloid-derived suppressor cell nomenclature and characterization standards. Nature Communications. 2016;**7**:12150

[41] Jin S, Yang Z, Hao X, Tang W, Ma W, Zong H. Roles of HMGB1 in regulating myeloid-derived suppressor cells in the tumor microenvironment. Biomarker Research. 2020;**8**:21

[42] Wu Y, Yi M, Niu M, Mei Q, Wu K. Myeloid-derived suppressor cells: An emerging target for anticancer immunotherapy. Molecular Cancer. 2022;**21**:184

[43] Nardo M, Reilley M, Biter A, Lim J, Bean SA, Nguyen LM, et al. Lefitolimod (TLR agonist) and ipilimumab in patients with advanced solid tumors: A phase I trial. Journal of Clinical Oncology [Internet]. 2023;**41**:2564. DOI: 10.1200/JCO.2023.41.16_suppl.2564

[44] Gandhi S, Opyrchal M, Grimm MJ, Slomba RT, Kokolus KM, Witkiewicz A, et al. Systemic infusion of TLR3-ligand and IFN-α in patients with breast cancer reprograms local tumor microenvironments for selective CTL influx. Journal for Immunotherapy of Cancer. 2023;**11**:e007381

[45] Trinh JQ, Acosta C, Easwar A, Galamaga R, Tan A. Durable and dramatic response to checkpoint inhibition combined with COX-2 inhibitor celecoxib in a patient with p16+ metastatic sinonasal undifferentiated carcinoma: A case

study. Cancer Reports. Hoboken, NJ, United States. 2024;7:e1915

[46] Scott EN, Gocher AM, Workman CJ, Vignali DAA. Regulatory T cells: Barriers of immune infiltration into the tumor microenvironment [Internet]. Frontiers in Immunology. 2021. DOI: 10.3389/fimmu.2021.702726

[47] Garon EB, Rizvi NA, Hui R, Leighl N, Balmanoukian AS, Eder JP, et al. Pembrolizumab for the treatment of non-small-cell lung cancer. The New England Journal of Medicine. 2015;**372**:2018-2028

[48] Ott PA, Bang Y-J, Piha-Paul SA, Razak ARA, Bennouna J, Soria J-C, et al. T-cell-inflamed gene-expression profile, programmed death ligand 1 expression, and tumor mutational burden predict efficacy in patients treated with Pembrolizumab across 20 cancers: KEYNOTE-028. Journal of Clinical Oncology: Official Journal of the American Society of Clinical Oncology. 2019;**37**:318-327

[49] Bagchi S, Yuan R, Engleman EG. Immune checkpoint inhibitors for the treatment of cancer: Clinical impact and mechanisms of response and resistance. Annual Review of Pathology. 2021;**16**:223-249

[50] Tay C, Tanaka A, Sakaguchi S. Tumor-infiltrating regulatory T cells as targets of cancer immunotherapy. Cancer Cell. 2023;**41**:450-465

[51] Shimizu J, Yamazaki S, Sakaguchi S. Induction of tumor immunity by removing CD25+CD4+ T cells: A common basis between tumor immunity and autoimmunity. Journal of Immunology. 1999;**163**:5211-5218

[52] Chan S, Belmar N, Ho S, Rogers B, Stickler M, Graham M, et al. An anti-PD-1-GITR-L bispecific agonist induces GITR clustering-mediated T cell activation for cancer immunotherapy. Nature Cancer. 2022;**3**:337-354

[53] Nishida N, Yano H, Nishida T, Kamura T, Kojiro M. Angiogenesis in cancer. Vascular Health and Risk Management. 2006;**2**:213-219

[54] Boere IA, Hamberg P, Sleijfer S. It takes two to tango: Combinations of conventional cytotoxics with compounds targeting the vascular endothelial growth factor-vascular endothelial growth factor receptor pathway in patients with solid malignancies. Cancer Science. 2010;**101**:7-15

[55] Vaupel P, Mayer A, Höckel M. Tumor hypoxia and malignant progression. Methods in Enzymology. 2004;**381**:335-354

[56] Casazza A, Di Conza G, Wenes M, Finisguerra V, Deschoemaeker S, Mazzone M. Tumor stroma: A complexity dictated by the hypoxic tumor microenvironment. Oncogene. 2014;**33**:1743-1754

[57] Wang B, Zhao Q, Zhang Y, Liu Z, Zheng Z, Liu S, et al. Targeting hypoxia in the tumor microenvironment: A potential strategy to improve cancer immunotherapy. Journal of Experimental & Clinical Cancer Research. 2021;**40**:24

[58] Bader JE, Voss K, Rathmell JC. Targeting metabolism to improve the tumor microenvironment for cancer immunotherapy. Molecular Cell. 2020;**78**:1019-1033

[59] Kim SW, Kim IK, Lee SH. Role of hyperoxic treatment in cancer. Experimental Biology and Medicine (Maywood, N.J.). 2020;**245**:851-860

[60] Chafe SC, McDonald PC, Saberi S, Nemirovsky O, Venkateswaran G,

Burugu S, et al. Targeting hypoxia-induced carbonic anhydrase IX enhances immune-checkpoint blockade locally and systemically. Cancer Immunology Research. 2019;**7**:1064-1078

[61] Spiegelberg L, Houben R, Niemans R, de Ruysscher D, Yaromina A, Theys J, et al. Hypoxia-activated prodrugs and (lack of) clinical progress: The need for hypoxia-based biomarker patient selection in phase III clinical trials. Clinical and Translational Radiation Oncology. 2019;**15**:62-69

[62] Zhong S, Jeong J-H, Chen Z, Chen Z, Luo J-L. Targeting tumor microenvironment by small-molecule inhibitors. Translational Oncology. 2020;**13**:57-69

[63] Baskar R, Lee KA, Yeo R, Yeoh K-W. Cancer and radiation therapy: Current advances and future directions. International Journal of Medical Sciences. 2012;**9**:193-199

[64] Nakajima S, Mimura K, Kaneta A, Saito K, Katagata M, Okayama H, et al. Radiation-induced remodeling of the tumor microenvironment through tumor cell-intrinsic expression of cGAS-STING in esophageal squamous cell carcinoma. International Journal of Radiation Oncology, Biology, Physics. 2023;**115**:957-971

[65] Lan Y, Moustafa M, Knoll M, Xu C, Furkel J, Lazorchak A, et al. Simultaneous targeting of TGF-β/PD-L1 synergizes with radiotherapy by reprogramming the tumor microenvironment to overcome immune evasion. Cancer Cell. 2021;**39**:1388-1403.e10

[66] Lin T, Zhang Q, Yuan A, Wang B, Zhang F, Ding Y, et al. Synergy of tumor microenvironment remodeling and autophagy inhibition to sensitize radiation for bladder cancer treatment. Theranostics. 2020;**10**:7683-7696

[67] Huang Y, Ruan Y, Ma Y, Chen D, Zhang T, Fan S, et al. Immunomodulatory activity of manganese dioxide nanoparticles: Promising for novel vaccines and immunotherapeutics. Frontiers in Immunology. 2023;**14**:1128840

[68] Wang L, Chard Dunmall LS, Cheng Z, Wang Y. Remodeling the tumor microenvironment by oncolytic viruses: Beyond oncolysis of tumor cells for cancer treatment. Journal for Immunotherapy of Cancer. 2022;**10**:e004167

[69] Samson A, West EJ, Carmichael J, Scott KJ, Turnbull S, Kuszlewicz B, et al. Neoadjuvant intravenous oncolytic vaccinia virus therapy promotes anticancer immunity in patients. Cancer Immunology Research. 2022;**10**:745-756

[70] Merrick AE, Ilett EJ, Melcher AA. JX-594, a targeted oncolytic poxvirus for the treatment of cancer. Current Opinion in Investigational Drugs. 2009;**10**:1372-1382

[71] Prestwich RJ, Harrington KJ, Pandha HS, Vile RG, Melcher AA, Errington F. Oncolytic viruses: A novel form of immunotherapy. Expert Review of Anticancer Therapy. 2008;**8**:1581-1588

[72] Guo ZS, Liu Z, Bartlett DL. Oncolytic immunotherapy: Dying the right way is a key to eliciting potent antitumor immunity. Frontiers in Oncology. 2014;**4**:74

[73] Merad M, Sathe P, Helft J, Miller J, Mortha A. The dendritic cell lineage: Ontogeny and function of dendritic cells and their subsets in the steady state and the inflamed setting. Annual Review of Immunology. 2013;**31**:563-604

[74] Gupta YH, Khanom A, Acton SE. Control of dendritic cell function within the tumour microenvironment. Frontiers in Immunology. 2022;**13**:733800

[75] Lopez MV, Rivera AA, Viale DL, Benedetti L, Cuneo N, Kimball KJ, et al. A tumor-stroma targeted oncolytic adenovirus replicated in human ovary cancer samples and inhibited growth of disseminated solid tumors in mice. Molecular Therapy. 2012;**20**:2222-2233

[76] Puig-Kröger A, Sierra-Filardi E, Domínguez-Soto A, Samaniego R, Corcuera MT, Gómez-Aguado F, et al. Folate receptor beta is expressed by tumor-associated macrophages and constitutes a marker for M2 anti-inflammatory/regulatory macrophages. Cancer Research. 2009;**69**:9395-9403

[77] Scott EM, Jacobus EJ, Lyons B, Frost S, Freedman JD, Dyer A, et al. Bi- and tri-valent T cell engagers deplete tumour-associated macrophages in cancer patient samples. Journal for Immunotherapy of Cancer. 2019;**7**:320

[78] Kaufman HL, Kohlhapp FJ, Zloza A. Oncolytic viruses: A new class of immunotherapy drugs. Nature Reviews. Drug Discovery. 2015;**14**:642-662

[79] Li Y-R, Dunn ZS, Yu Y, Li M, Wang P, Yang L. Advancing cell-based cancer immunotherapy through stem cell engineering. Cell Stem Cell. 2023;**30**:592-610

[80] Pickup MW, Mouw JK, Weaver VM. The extracellular matrix modulates the hallmarks of cancer. EMBO Reports. 2014;**15**:1243-1253

[81] Schaaf MB, Garg AD, Agostinis P. Defining the role of the tumor vasculature in antitumor immunity and immunotherapy. Cell Death & Disease. 2018;**9**:115

[82] Tie Y, Tang F, Wei Y-Q, Wei X-W. Immunosuppressive cells in cancer: Mechanisms and potential therapeutic targets. Journal of Hematology & Oncology. 2022;**15**:61

[83] Sterner RC, Sterner RM. CAR-T cell therapy: Current limitations and potential strategies. Blood Cancer Journal. 2021;**11**:69

[84] Sanber K, Savani B, Jain T. Graft-versus-host disease risk after chimeric antigen receptor T-cell therapy: The diametric opposition of T cells. British Journal of Haematology. 2021;**195**:660-668

[85] Lv M, Wang K, Huang X-J. Myeloid-derived suppressor cells in hematological malignancies: Friends or foes. Journal of Hematology & Oncology. 2019;**12**:105

[86] Caruana I, Savoldo B, Hoyos V, Weber G, Liu H, Kim ES, et al. Heparanase promotes tumor infiltration and antitumor activity of CAR-redirected T lymphocytes. Nature Medicine. 2015;**21**:524-529

[87] John LB, Devaud C, Duong CPM, Yong CS, Beavis PA, Haynes NM, et al. Anti-PD-1 antibody therapy potently enhances the eradication of established tumors by gene-modified T cells. Clinical Cancer Research: An Official Journal of the American Association for Cancer Research. 2013;**19**:5636-5646

[88] Grosser R, Cherkassky L, Chintala N, Adusumilli PS. Combination immunotherapy with CAR T cells and checkpoint blockade for the treatment of solid Tumors. Cancer Cell. 2019;**36**:471-482

[89] He X, Xu C. Immune checkpoint signaling and cancer immunotherapy. Cell Research. 2020;**30**:660-669

Chapter 4

Colony-Stimulating Factor 1 Receptor: A Novel Target for Cancer Immunotherapy

Jiachen Wen, Shenglin Luan and Dan Liu

Abstract

The Colony-Stimulating Factor 1 (CSF-1) and its receptor (CSF1R) constitute an important axis that regulates the phenotype of most tissue-resident macrophages. Endogenous cytokine ligation and oncogenic mutations of CSF1R trigger the activation of several downstream pro-survival kinase cascades, thereby enhancing tumor cell proliferation and disease progression. Tumor-associate macrophages (TAMs) harboring activated CSF1R release tumorigenic cytokines, thus further deconditioning tumor immune microenvironment to a pro-tumoral phenotype. With the recent success of pexidartinib for the treatment of tenosynovial giant cell tumor, CSF1R pathway blockage has emerged as a promising TAM-targeting approach in certain types of cancers. More interventions to CSF1R, including monotherapy and combinatorial therapy, have advanced to clinical trials for a broader spectrum of cancers, highlighting such strategy to benefit cancer immunotherapy.

Keywords: colony-stimulating factor 1 receptor, receptor tyrosine kinase, tumor-associated macrophages, tumor microenvironment, immunotherapy

1. Introduction

Colony-Stimulating Factor 1 Receptor (CSF1R) is a transmembrane receptor tyrosine kinase (RTK) that is activated by two cognate cytokines, Colony-Stimulating Factor-1 (CSF-1) and Interleukin-34 (IL-34) [1, 2]. Following their binding to the ectodomain of CSF1R, the topology of the resulting protein complex proved to be discrepant [3]. The topological discrepancy may translate into several distinct yet overlapping downstream effects. Conclusively, the binding of either ligand induces CSF1R dimerization and releases of the intracellular tyrosine kinase from an autoinhibitory state [4, 5]. Kinase activation further triggers the recruitment of several downstream effector proteins, including PI3K, JAK, and MAPKs, whose activations are essential for cell survival, proliferation, and differentiation [6].

CSF1R is abundantly expressed in myeloid cells, including macrophages, microglial cells, and dendritic cells, but low in myeloid precursor cells [7–9]. Macrophages constitute an important part of the innate and adaptive immunity and are essential components of the inflammatory microenvironment of diseased tissues [10]. Diseases like cancers could annex the immune system to promote disease progression [11]. As critical members of the tumor microenvironment (TME), tissue-resident macrophages and monocyte-derived cells are prone to be recruited to the hypoxic or necrotic areas of tumor tissues, where they may further differentiate into tumor-associated macrophages (TAMs) influenced by various stimulation factors [11]. In certain cases, accumulated tumor-infiltrating TAMs could even reach more than half of the tumor weight, and these often relate to poor prognosis and chemoresistance [12]. In response to TME perturbations, TAMs demonstrate a broad spectrum of homeostatic status [12]. Of which, the M1-like and M2-like statuses represent two polarized forms of TAMs (**Figure 1**) [12]. The M1-like macrophages promote immune-mediated tumor suppression through the release of proinflammatory cytokines (IL-1β, IL-6, and TNF-α), whereas the M2-like macrophages demonstrate pro-tumoral activity in many ways, including immunosuppression, promoting angiogenesis, and abundant secretion of tumorigenic cytokines [13]. In response to the TME primed by multifunctional cytokines, M1-like macrophages often tend to shift toward an M2-like phenotype, where the activation of CSF1R plays a vital role throughout the process [14].

Blockage of the CSF-1/CSF1R axis to prevent the recruitment and transformation of M2-like TAMs is an attractive yet the only truly selective approach for TAM manipulation [15]. In the past few years, CSF1R inhibition has been reported to

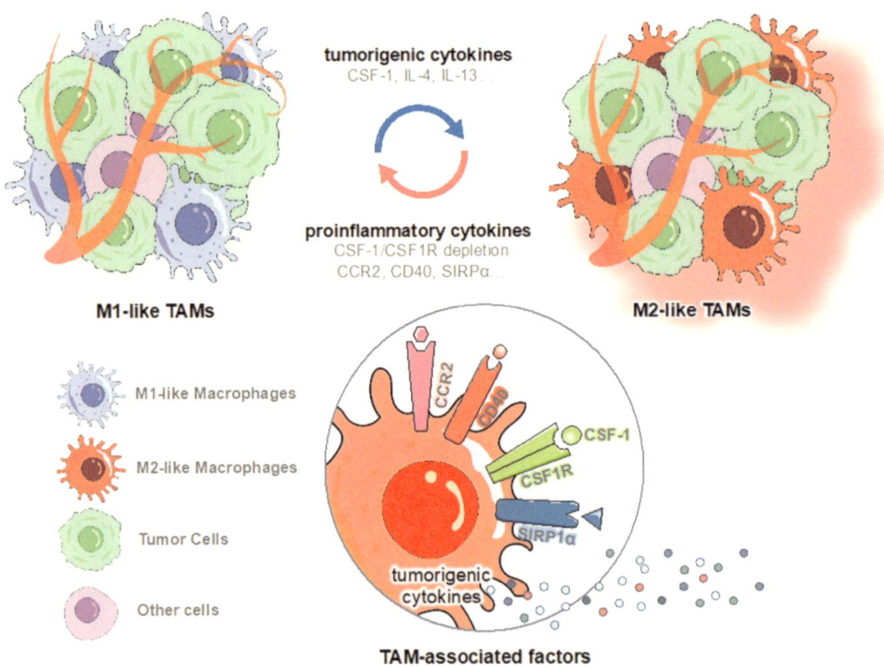

Figure 1.
CSF-1/CSF1R regulate TME. Interconverted model of M1-like macrophages and M2-like macrophages. CSF1R and other transmembrane receptors expressed on macrophages, once been activated, could release tumorigenic cytokines, including CCL2, IL-6, and IL-10, thus further deconditioning TME.

fascinatingly repolarize M2-like toward M1-like TAMs and block tumor progression in various preclinical and clinical settings [15]. It is worth to note that many studies favored the therapeutic role of CSF1R depleting, including glioblastoma (GBM) [16], medulloblastoma [17], malignant meningiomas [18], colorectal cancer [19], hematologic malignancies [20], and notably tenosynovial giant cell tumor (TGCT) [10]. Beyond tumors abundantly expressing CSF1R, pharmaceutically targeting CSF1R may also reform TME in CSF1R-less abundant tumors [21]. Nevertheless, controversial results have been observed in certain cases. A recently disclosed phase II trial regarding CSF1R inhibitor (pexidartinib) for recurrent GBM patients showed no statistically significant overall response, albeit two patients of which showed extended survival [22]. Since clinically distinct GBM subtypes exist, it is plausible that different patients diversify their responses to CSF1R-targeted therapy.

CSF1R is composed of 972 amino acids [6]. The molecular weight of a mature protein is around 110 to 165 kDa due to varying degrees of glycosylation [6]. As a multidomain protein, CSF1R consists of an extracellular domain (aa1–512), an intracellular domain (aa538–972), and a single transmembrane segment (aa513–537) (**Figure 2**) [6]. The extracellular domain can be further specified as five immunoglobulin (Ig) domains and a linker region. It has been reported that the first three Igs (D1–D3) confer ligand

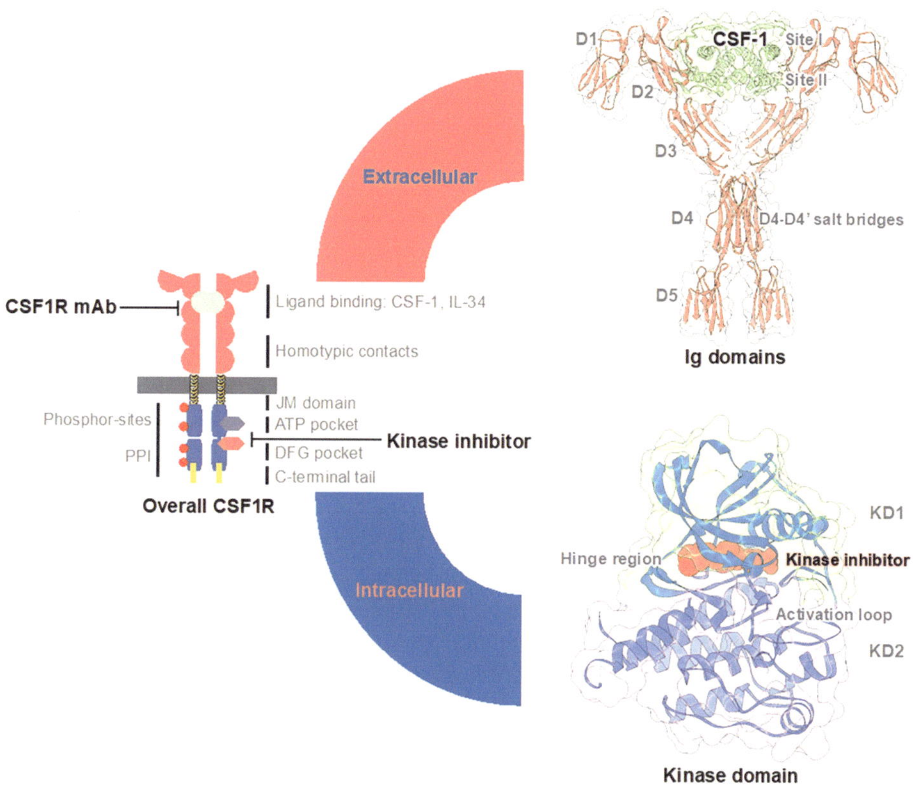

Figure 2.
Structure of CSF1R. Following binding of CSF-1 to the Ig domains, CSF1R dimerization initiates KD autophosphorylation. Crystal structures demonstrate CSF-1 in complexed with the Ig domains (PDB ID: 4WRM and 4WRL) and the KD domain complexed with pexidartinib (PDB ID: 4R7H), which provide distinct drug-binding sites for CSF1R modulating. All structures are prepared through UCSF chimera [23].

recognition, whereas D4–D5 stabilize the ligand and the ligand-induced dimerization [24]. The intracellular domain consists of a juxtamembrane (JM) domain, a kinase domain (KD), and a C-terminal tail [6]. The KD is interrupted by a flexible hinge sequence, thereafter generating KD1 and KD2 modules [6]. The KD1 anchors the ATP, whereas the KD2 mediates substrate binding.

Strategies have been proposed to modulate functions of this multidomain protein. Monoclonal antibodies targeting the Ig domains of CSF1R could generally prevent the CSF-1/CSF1R recognition and CSF1R dimerization, and thereafter KD activation [24]. Emactuzumab may represent the first clinically investigated CSF1R-targeting antibody [24]. A phase III study of emactuzumab has been initiated to assess the efficacy and safety in subjects with TGCT (NCT05417789). This study focuses on patients with localized or diffused type TGCT where surgical removal of the tumor is not optional. On the other hand, kinase inhibitors targeting the KD of CSF1R may generally prevent itself from transactivation and cytosolic signaling transduction [22]. Pexidartinib is a small-molecule, orally available kinase inhibitor with selective activity against CSF1R, KIT, and FLT3-ITD [25]. In 2019, pexidartinib has been approved by the FDA for TGCT patients associated with severe morbidity or functional limitation and not amenable for surgery [25].

Encouraged by the approval of pexidartinib, CSF1R emerged early on as a promising immunotherapeutic target. A number of structurally diversified small-molecule inhibitors and therapeutic antibodies have been proposed in the past few years for TGCT treatment and beyond [26]. In the following section, we have brought together the ever-growing advances of CSF1R-targeting antagonists advanced to clinic, including small-molecule inhibitors and therapeutic antibodies.

2. Small-molecule CSF1R inhibitors

Dozens of CSF1R inhibitors have advanced to clinical trials, with more than 10 oncology programs actively recruiting now (https://clinicaltrials.gov, data accessed Nov. 2023). In **Table 1**, we have summarized the clinical hallmarks of these CSF1R drugs (candidates) one by one, with their chemical structures illustrated in **Figure 3**. Notably, as a member of the tyrosine kinase family, several approved drugs more or less involve CSF1R inhibition, including imatinib and dasatinib. We will not include those drugs as their therapeutic effects under functioning concentrations are mostly CSF1R independent [27].

2.1 PLX3397 (Pexidartinib)

Pexidartinib (Plexxikon) is the first FDA-approved CSF1R inhibitor for TGCT management [28]. It potently inhibited CSF1R (IC_{50} = 17 nM) and two other evolutionary-related kinases, c-KIT (12 nM) and FLT3 (9 nM) [28]. ENLIVEN is a randomized, multinational phase III trial for pexidartinib (NCT02371369). Throughout the study, 5% of recipients had a complete response and 51% had a partial response [28]. Pexidartinib also improved patient symptoms and physical functional outcomes in ENLIVEN. Unfortunately, another trial against recurrent GBM failed to demonstrate efficacy, even adequate drug exposure being confirmed (NCT01349036). Correlative studies are warranted to test the hypothesis of how the relative proportion of GBM subtypes could have resulted in treatment resistance [29]. It is worth noting that pexidartinib includes a boxed warning on the risk

Drug	Highest clinical stage	Indication	References
Pexidartinib	Approved	TGCT PVNS GIST PAAD/COAD SKCM GBM Solid tumors	NCT04488822 NCT02371369 NCT03158103 (w/ Binimetinib) NCT02777710 (w/ Durvalumab) NCT02975700 NCT01349036 NCT01525602 (w/ Paclitaxel)
Sulfatinib	Approved	NET THCA OS BTC CRC NSCLC HCC HNSC GIST TNBC OC Solid tumors	NCT02588170 NCT02614495 NCT05590572 NCT03873532 NCT05372198 NCT04922658 NCT05282433 NCT04910854 NCT05030246 (w/ Toripalimab) NCT05746728 (w/ Tislelizumab) NCT05652283 (w/ Pamiparib) NCT04169672
DCC-3014	III	TGCT SARC	NCT05059262 NCT04242238
ABSK021	III	TGCT PDAC Solid tumors	NCT05804045 NCT06111274 (w/ Chemotherapy) NCT04192344
JNJ-40346527	II	AML PRAD HL RA	NCT03557970 NCT03177460 NCT01572519 NCT01597739
BLZ945	II	Solid tumors	NCT02829723
ARRY-382	I/II	Solid tumors	NCT01316822 NCT02880371 (w/ Pembrolizumab)
NMS-088	I/II	AML/CMML	NCT03922100
Q702	I/II	Solid tumors	NCT04648254 NCT05438420 (w/ Pembrolizumab)
TPX-0022	I/II	Solid tumors	NCT03993873
PLX73086	I	TGCT	NCT02673736
PLX7486	I	Solid tumors	NCT01804530
SYHA1813	I	Solid tumors	ChiCTR2100045380

Table 1.
CSF1R-targeting chemical drugs in clinical trials.

of serious and potentially fatal liver injury, highlighting the continuous need for new drug investigation [28].

2.2 HMPL-012 (Sulfatinib)

Sulfatinib (Hutchmed), an oral angio-immuno kinase inhibitor, has been approved for the use of extrapancreatic neuroendocrine tumors (NET) in China [30].

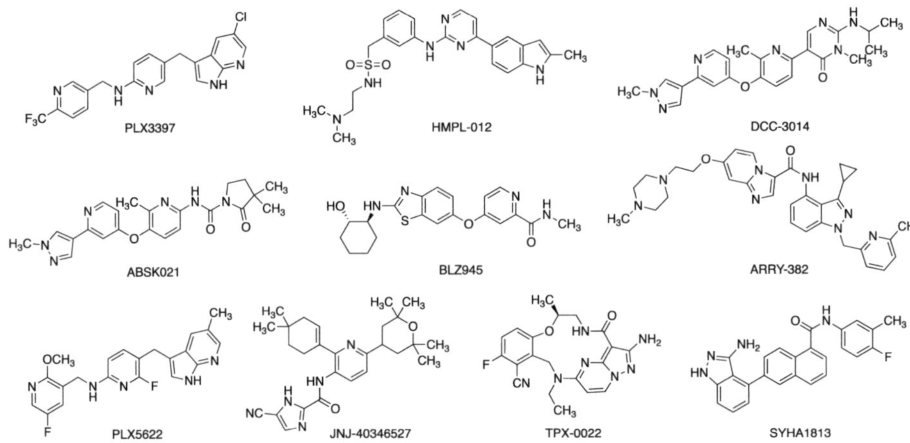

Figure 3.
Structures of CSF1R inhibitors advanced to clinical trials.

It selectively targets CSF1R (IC_{50} = 4 nM), VEGFR1–3 (1–24 nM), and FGFR1 (15 nM) while weakly inhibiting 278 other kinases (IC_{50} > 150 nM) [30]. SANET-ep is a randomized, double-blind, multicenter phase III trial, in which surufatinib prolonged progression-free survival in Chinese patients with advanced extrapancreatic NET (NCT02588170). A recent phase II trial demonstrated surufatinib in combination with toripalimab (an anti-PD-1 antibody) for locally advanced thyroid cancer was feasible, and the majority of patients achieved R0 resection (NCT04524884) [31].

2.3 DCC-3014 (Vimseltinib)

Deciphera Pharmaceuticals has recently proposed a potent CSF1R inhibitor (DCC-3014), with an IC_{50} of 2.2 nM [32]. DCC-3014 demonstrated improved selectivity over pexidartinib and favorable drug-like properties [32]. Three trials ranging from phase I to III are currently underway (NCT03069469, NCT04242238, NCT05059262). Early disclosed phase I data suggested DCC-3014 solely or in combination with avelumab (anti-PD-L1 antibody) was generally safe and tolerable in patients with advanced tumors [33]. In patients bearing TGCT, DCC-3014 showed encouraging antitumor activity with an overall objective response rate (ORR) of 42% [34]. Very recently, a phase III trial (MOTION) carried out to access the effectiveness of DCC-3014 in inoperable TGCT patients (NCT05059262).

2.4 ABSK021 (Pimicotinib)

ABSK021 (Abbisko Therapeutics) has potent biochemical and cellular activities against CSF1R (IC_{50} < 30 nM) and over 40-fold selectivity against c-KIT, FLT3, PDGFR, and VEGFR2 [35]. Recently disclosed phase I study supported ABSK021 to be further evaluated in advanced solid tumors, as optimistic safety profile and having favorable PK/PD properties [36]. Phase Ib study furthered the conclusion that ABSK021 has significant antitumor activity in TGCT patients, with no apparent hepatotoxicity [37]. MANEUVER is a randomized, double-blind, placebo-controlled, multicenter phase III study to assess the efficacy and safety of ABSK021 in patients with TGCT (NCT05804045). Very recently, a phase II trial has launched to assess the efficacy and safety of ABSK021 in combination with chemotherapy with or without toripalimab in patients with advanced pancreatic cancer (PDAC) (NCT06111274).

2.5 JNJ-40346527 (Edicotinib)

Johnson Pharmaceuticals proposed their CSF1R candidates, with JNJ-40346527 exhibiting potent CSF1R inhibition (IC_{50} = 3.2 nM) and selectivity over c-KIT and FLT3 [38]. Clinical trial of JNJ-40346527 is ongoing in patients with certain types of prostate cancer (NCT03177460). Another trial in patients with relapsed or refractory (R/R) acute myeloid leukemia (AML) was terminated in 2021 due to not enough enrollment (NCT03557970). Unfortunately, JNJ-40346527 demonstrated limited efficacy in patients with R/R Hodgkin lymphoma (HL) when administered solely (NCT01572519).

2.6 BLZ945 (Sotuletinib)

BLZ945 (Novartis) is an orally active, brain-penetrable CSF1R inhibitor with outstanding potency (IC_{50} = 1 nM) and selectivity (above 3200-fold selectivity over kinases) [39]. The study of BLZ945 in patients with advanced solid tumors has decided to terminate without disclosed details (NCT02829723). However, early disclosed results suggested BLZ945 alone or in combination with spartalizumab (anti-PD-1 antibody) was safety acceptable [40].

2.7 ARRY-382 (PF-07265804)

ARRY-382 (Pfizer) is a highly selective, orally available CSF1R inhibitor (IC_{50} = 9 nM), with no significant inhibition against c-KIT and PDGFR [41]. Phase I study in patients with advanced solid tumors has established MTD and RP2D [41]. Favorable PK and partial response were observed through the regimen (NCT01316822). A phase I/II study of ARRY-382 in combination with pembrolizumab (anti-PD-1 antibody) for the treatment of patients with advanced solid tumors was initiated in 2016 (NCT02880371). However, the trial was halted in 2022 for the reason of insufficient efficacy [42].

2.8 NMS-088

NMS-088 (Nerviano Medical Sciences) is a brain-penetrable CSF1R, c-KIT, and FLT3 triple inhibitor, with Kd values below 1 nM for all three targets [43]. NMS-088 is currently being evaluated clinically in patients with R/R AML or chronic myelomonocytic leukemia (CMML) (NCT03922100). In the ongoing phase I/II study, NMS-088 showed manageable safety with no MTD being reached [44]. NMS-088 demonstrated dose-dependent clinical responses in FLT3 positive R/R AML patients, including patients who have failed prior FLT3 inhibitors [44]. Pharmacokinetic profile also showed proportional increase with the dose [44]. These results warrant further development of NMS-088 as a potential therapeutic option for patients who have exhausted available treatments.

2.9 Q702

Q702 (Qurient Therapeutics) is an orally available CSF1R, Axl, and Mer triple inhibitor, and is developed to modulate innate TME [45]. Q702 is currently under two clinical trials. One phase I study aims to establish safety, tolerability, and PK/PD profile in patients with advanced solid tumors (NCT04648254). The other phase I/II clinical trial seeks to determine safety and preliminary efficacy of Q702 in combination with anti-PD-1 therapy in patients with advanced solid tumors (NCT05438420). Preliminary data suggested Q702 demonstrated the intended pharmacologic activity with acceptable safety profile [46].

2.10 TPX-0022 (Elzovantinib)

TPX-0022 (Turning Point Therapeutics) is a potent CSF1R (IC_{50} = 0.76 nM), MET, and Src triple inhibitor [47]. Study of TPX-0022 is currently underway in patients with advanced solid tumors harboring genetic alterations in MET (NCT03993873). Early disclosed data from this phase I/II trial suggested TPX-0022 was well-tolerated [48].

2.11 PLX5622

Aiming to develop novel CSF1R-selective inhibitors that are able to achieve robust brain-wide microglia elimination, Plexxikon further developed a series of drug candidates based on the existing pexidartinib [49]. PLX5622 exhibited strong affinity to CSF1R (IC_{50} = 16 nM) and improved brain penetrance [49]. Unlike pexidartinib, it possesses higher selectivity over c-KIT and FLT3 at above 20-fold [49]. Plus, no inhibition was observed against over 230 other kinases at 1 μM. PLX5622 has advanced to clinical trial for safety, tolerability, and PK evaluation in healthy adults (NCT01282684).

In the meanwhile, two other CSF1R inhibitors have also marched to clinic. PLX73086 is a potent and selective CSF1R inhibitor targeting TAMs [50]. A phase I trial of PLX73086 in patients with advanced solid tumors and R/R TGCT was initiated in 2016 (NCT02673736). Besides, as the first CSF1R/Trk dual inhibitor, PLX7486 has entered phase I trial in patients with advanced solid tumors (NCT01804530).

2.12 SYHA1813

SYHA1813 (CSPC Pharmaceutical) is a CSF1R (IC_{50} = 19.3 nM), VEGFR1 ~ 3 (IC_{50} = 0.3 ~ 4.3 nM) dual inhibitor able to penetrate the blood-brain barrier [51]. It has advanced to phase I trial in China in patients with recurrent high-grade gliomas (HGG) or advanced solid tumors (ChiCTR2100045380). Preliminary data suggested oral administration of SYHA1813 at 15 mg/day was acceptable and active in recurrent HGG [52]. Later dose-expansion results demonstrated encouraging ORR with a well-tolerated safety profile in patients with recurrent meningioma [53].

3. CSF1R-targeting monoclonal antibodies

CSF1R-targeting antibodies offer the possibility to treat tumors in a targeted fashion and reduce the side effects often roused by promiscuous kinase inhibitors [54]. In a way similar to the endogenous ligands CSF-1 and IL-34, most of the clinically investigated CSF1R-targeting antibodies recognize the first three Igs (D1–D3), thus preventing the formation of ligand/receptor complex (**Table 2**) [55]. Additionally, few antibodies bind to D4–D5 that blocks the dimerization interface of CSF1R [55]. Unlike the recent success of small-molecule inhibitors, current leading CSF1R-targeting antibody programs struggled in several oncology settings [55].

Drug	Highest clinical stage	Indication	Reference
Emactuzumab	III	TGCT Solid tumors	NCT05417789 NCT02323191 (w/Atezolizumab) NCT02760797 (w/Selicrelumab) NCT01494688 (w/Paclitaxel)
FPA008	II	TGCT PTCL HCC BTC PDAC Solid tumors	NCT02471716 NCT03927105 (w/Nivolumab) NCT04050462 (w/Nivolumab) NCT03768531 (w/Nivolumab) NCT03336216 (w/Nivolumab) NCT02526017 (w/Nivolumab)
LY3022855	II	BC MM Solid tumors	NCT02265536 NCT03101254 (w/Vemurafenib) NCT01346358 NCT02718911 (w/Durvalumab)
SNDX-6352	II	iCCA HL	NCT04301778 (w/Durvalumab) NCT05723055 (w/Nivolumab)
AMB-05X	II	TGCT	NCT05349643
AMG 820	I/II	Solid tumors	NCT01444404 NCT02713529 (w/Pembrolizumab)

Table 2.
CSF1R-targeting biological drugs in clinical trials.

3.1 RG7155 (Emactuzumab)

The emactuzumab monoclonal antibody (Roche) inhibits CSF1R (IC_{50} = 0.3 nM), causing cell death and reducing CD68/CD163 macrophages [56]. In a previously disclosed phase I trial in patients with advanced solid tumors, emactuzumab showed clinical activity in locally advanced or relapsed TGCT and was associated with a manageable safety profile (NCT01494688). Tumor responses were durable, and most patients had profound symptomatic and functional improvement. It is also currently under a phase III (TANGENT) study to further access the efficacy and safety in TGCT patients (NCT05417789). A recent disclosed phase 1b study suggested emactuzumab in combination with atezolizumab (anti-PD-L1 antibody) was generally safe, with a considerable ORR observed in non-small cell lung cancer (NSCLC) patients (NCT02323191) [57].

3.2 FPA008 (Cabiralizumab)

FPA008 (FivePrime) is a monoclonal antibody against CSF1R and is currently under phase II trial for TGCT treatment [58]. In 2017, preliminary data of a phase I/II study of FPA008 suggested positive functional status improvements (NCT02471716). FPA008 is currently being evaluated in a collection of clinical settings, mostly in combination with anti-PD-1 therapy, to target immune cells, macrophages, and monocytes in advanced solid tumors [55].

3.3 LY3022855

LY3022855 (Eli Lilly) is a recombinant human monoclonal antibody that prevents binding of CSF-1 and IL-34 to CSF1R [59]. A previous phase I study of LY3022855 monotherapy in patients with metastatic breast cancer (BC) demonstrated good tolerability and target engagement activity, with two patients achieving stable disease for over 9 months (NCT02265536) [60]. However, LY3022855 combined with durvalumab (anti-PD-L1 antibody) or tremelimumab (anti-CTLA-4 antibody) in patients with advanced NSCLC or ovarian cancer (OC) had limited clinical activity [55]. LY3022855 in combination with BRAF/MEK inhibition was difficult to tolerate in a small melanoma (MM) population [61]. One response was observed in this small sample of patients, suggesting this combination might be worthy of further exploration [61].

3.4 SNDX-6352 (Axatilimab)

SNDX-6352 (Syndax Pharmaceuticals) is a humanized antibody of high CSF1R-binding affinity [62]. SNDX-6352 affects the migration, proliferation, differentiation, and survival of monocytes and macrophages by binding to CSF1R and blocking its activation [62]. Several clinical trials of SNDX-6352 solely or in combination in patients with solid tumors are underway [55]. Particularly, the combination of SNDX-6352 and anti-PD-L1 therapy was generally well tolerated in patients with advanced intrahepatic cholangiocarcinoma (iCCA), plus some signal of activity observed [63].

3.5 AMB-05X

AMB-05X (AmMax Bio) is a fully humanized antibody targeting CSF1R in development for local treatment of TGCT [64]. Intra-articular injection of AMB-05X enables high drug concentration at the tumor site while minimizing systemic exposure and toxicity [64]. Recently disclosed phase I data of AMB-05X found clinically meaningful improvement in ORR and quality of life measures after 12 weeks of therapy, with a limited number of adverse events [64]. The ongoing phase II study aims to establish the dosing regimen of AMB-05X and confirm the efficacy and safety of 24 weeks and longer treatment (NCT05349643).

3.6 AMG 820

AMG 820 (AmMax Bio) is another CSF1R-targeting antibody that inhibits binding of CSF-1 and IL-34 and subsequent receptor activation [65]. Preclinically, AMG 820 potently inhibited CSF-1-driven proliferation of human bone marrow–derived monocytic [65]. In phase I study in patients with advanced solid tumors, AMG 820 was tolerated with manageable toxicities [65]. PD response was demonstrated, despite limited antitumor activity observed (NCT01444404). A follow-up phase Ib/II study has been carried out to assess the safety and anti-tumor activity of AMG 820 in combination with anti-PD-1 therapy, with no result disclosed yet (NCT02713529).

4. CSF1R-targeting agents as combinatorial therapy

Despite the success of CSF1R inhibitors in the management of TGCT, studies in other oncology settings are mostly up the creek. Coincidentally, CSF1R inhibition barely slowed tumor progression in a set of preclinical models but rarely led to tumor regression [26]. It is argued that the lack of efficacy is in part by the fact that long-term tumor control requires active engagement of the adaptive immune system, which might not be fully triggered by TAM-targeting agents [66]. Conversely, tumors often resist chemotherapy, radiation therapy, and immunotherapy by secreting CSF-1, an important tumorigenic cytokine [26]. Many possibilities implying CSF1R inhibitors better serve as combinatorial agents to migrate the immunosuppression and potentiate tumor response [26]. As a consequence, multiple trials evaluating CSF1R inhibitors in combination are currently underway (referring to **Tables 1** and **2**).

4.1 Combination with immune-checkpoint inhibitors

Immune-checkpoint inhibitors (ICIs) represent a significant breakthrough in oncology immunotherapy. Instead of killing the tumor cells directly, their antitumor effects are generally mediated by the activation of antitumoral T cells [67, 68]. Activated $CD8^+$ T cells secrete several pro-tumoral cytokines, including TNF-α and IFN-γ, thereafter further inducing the expression of CSF-1 [11]. The activated CSF-1/CSF1R axis in turn facilitates TAM infiltration, inducing an immunosuppressive and pro-tumoral TME [12]. Consequently, the concomitant blockade of the CSF1R axis and immune checkpoint system may function in a synergistical manner [69].

Several combinations of CSF1R inhibition with anti-PD-1, anti-PD-L1, or anti-CTLA-4 therapies have advanced to the clinic (referring to **Tables 1** and **2**). More than 10 studies have finished their phase I investigation, with most results demonstrating well tolerability [26]. Several advanced trials further proved their initial efficacy against various tumoral settings [26]. Notably, emactuzumab in combination with anti-PD-L1 antibody (atezolizumab) demonstrated a considerable ORR in ICB-experienced NSCLC patients. An increase of $CD8^+$ T cells under therapy appeared to be associated with the persistence of a TAM subpopulation [57].

4.2 Combination with chemotherapy

Several studies implying chemotherapeutic agents may enhance TAMs' presence in cancers [70]. In patients with breast cancer, a higher percentage of $CD45^+$ $CD11b^+$ $CD14^+$ macrophages is observed in patients who receive chemotherapy. Elevated TAMs in turn suppress the cytotoxic effects of chemotherapies [71]. In preclinical models, TAM depletion with CSF1R inhibitor potentiates the efficacy of paclitaxel, an important first-line medication against a collection of solid tumors [71].

Clinically, pexidartinib or emactuzumab in combination with paclitaxel in tumor patients demonstrated well-tolerability and PD responsiveness [72]. Particularly, the pexidartinib group demonstrated 16% full or partial response and 34% stable disease [72]. A study for pexidartinib and rapamycin combination is underway (NCT02584647). Phase I data suggested safety and preliminary effectiveness, including 17% partial responses and 50% stable disease [73].

4.3 Combination with targeted therapy

In spite of high initial efficacy, targeted therapies hardly cure cancers before they develop resistance. Acquired resistance to olaparib (a PARP inhibitor) has been observed in *BRCA1*-deficient metaplastic breast cancer [74]. Mechanism study suggested PARP inhibition modulates the TME in *BRCA1*-deficient triple-negative breast cancer (TNBC) and results in TAM infiltration [75]. CSF1R inhibition reduced the population of immunosuppressive macrophage and overcame resistance in *BRCA1*-deficient TNBC [75]. As a consequence, combining PARP inhibitor with anti-CSF1R antibody significantly enhanced innate and adaptive antitumor immunity and extended survival in mice bearing *BRCA*-deficient tumors [75].

Pexidartinib was found to significantly block tumor progression in a PDGFB-driven GBM mouse model [76]. Interestingly, the multitargeted tyrosine kinase inhibitors dovitinib and vatalanib only exerted minimal efficacy [76]. TME alteration by CSF1R inhibition rendered tumor cells more susceptible to tyrosine kinase inhibition in preclinical models, which may have important translational relevance [76]. A phase I study of pexidartinib in combination with vemurafenib ($BRAF^{V600E}$ inhibitor) has been initiated in patients with MM (NCT01826448). Preliminary data suggested well-tolerability, with no serious adverse events observed [26]. A subsequent study of binimetinib (MEK inhibitor) in combination with pexidartinib in advanced gastrointestinal stromal tumor (GIST) demonstrated well-tolerability, with meaningful clinical response observed in two imatinib-refractory patients (NCT03158103). Moreover, a phase I/II trial of PLX9486 in combination with pexidartinib or sunitinib in participants with advanced solid tumors was well-tolerated, with evidence of activity against GIST [77].

5. Conclusions

TAM manipulation has been acknowledged as an attractive antitumor strategy. This could be further specified into inhibition of TAM recruitment, repolarization of TAMs, or direct depletion of TAMs. Among numerous TAM-related mechanisms, CSF-1/CSF1R, CCR2, CCR5, CD47/SIRP1α, CXCL12/CXCR4, and TERM-targeting antagonists, as well as CD40, ANG2, and TLR-targeting agonists have advanced to the clinic [78]. Unlike many receptors only expressed in a limited subset of TAMs, CSF1R is prevalently present in almost every type of TAMs. Pharmacological inhibition CSF1R has emerged as an immunotherapy to reduce TAM population, especially the pro-tumoral, immunosuppressive M2-like TAMs.

Small molecules and therapeutic antibodies are two concurrent methodologies targeting CSF1R. Significant progress has been achieved in the past few years, particularly in the field of TGCT management. However, some fundamental questions remain to be addressed [26]. Developing CSF1R-selective inhibitors that are devoid of RTK III family inhibition is challenging, as c-KIT and FLT3 share strong sequence similarity to CSF1R. Benefitting from the acquired crystal models, researchers have developed a number of structural diversified drug candidates that largely fulfilled the chemical space of CSF1R inhibitors. Compounds bearing 2-(1-methyl-1*H*-pyrazol-4-yl) pyridine, benzo [*d*] thiazole, imidazo [1,2-*a*] pyridine, 1*H*-pyrrolo [2,3-*b*] pyridine building blocks have demonstrated outstanding CSF1R-selectivity among RTK III family in preclinical settings.

Current immunotherapies, represented by ICIs and adoptive cell therapy, rely on reinforcing endogenous cytotoxic $CD8^+$ T cells to durably control tumors in some patients. The establishment of these immunotherapies are revolutionizing but only benefit a small proportion of patients. It is urgent to know if novel therapeutic targets could be identified within the multifarious TME. In this chapter, we concluded CSF1R as a novel target for cancer immunotherapy. Through manipulating macrophages, CSF1R-targeting therapies have demonstrated initial success and are expected to further expand the landscape of immunotherapy to a broader field.

Acknowledgements

We appreciate the Basic Research Program of Educational Commission of Liaoning Province of China (JYTQN2023322) and the Youth Talent Project of Shenyang Pharmaceutical University (YQ202207) to support this work.

Conflict of interest

The authors declare no conflict of interest.

Author details

Jiachen Wen[1*], Shenglin Luan[2] and Dan Liu[1]

1 Key Laboratory of Structure-Based Drugs Design and Discovery of Ministry of Education, Shenyang Pharmaceutical University, Shenyang, China

2 China Resources Sanjiu Medical and Pharmaceutical Co., Ltd, Shenzhen, China

*Address all correspondence to: wenjiachen@syphu.edu.cn

References

[1] Rojo R, Raper A, Ozdemir DD, et al. Deletion of a Csf1r enhancer selectively impacts CSF1R expression and development of tissue macrophage populations. Nature Communications. 2019;**10**:3215. DOI: 10.1038/s41467-019-11053-8

[2] Sehgal A, Donaldson DS, Pridans C, et al. The role of CSF1R-dependent macrophages in control of the intestinal stem-cell niche. Nature Communications. 2018;**9**:1272. DOI: 10.1038/s41467-018-03638-6

[3] Sehgal A, Irvine KM, Hume DA. Functions of macrophage colony-stimulating factor (CSF1) in development, homeostasis, and tissue repair. Seminars in Immunology. 2021;**54**:101509. DOI: 10.1016/j.smim.2021.101509

[4] Walter M, Lucet IS, Patel O, et al. The 2.7 Å crystal structure of the autoinhibited human c-FMS kinase domain. Journal of Molecular Biology. 2007;**367**:839-847. DOI: 10.1016/j.jmb.2007.01.036

[5] Ayudhya CCN, Graidist P, Tipmanee V. Potential stereoselective binding of trans-(±)-Kusunokinin and cis-(±)-Kusunokinin isomers to CSF1R. Molecules. 2022;**27**:4194. DOI: 10.3390/molecules27134194

[6] Stanley ER, Chitu V. CSF-1 receptor signaling in myeloid cells. Cold Spring Harbor in Perspectives in Biology. 2014;**6**:a021857. DOI: 10.1101/cshperspect.a021857

[7] Wilhelmsen K, van der Geer P. Phorbol 12-myristate 13-acetate-induced release of the colony-stimulating factor 1 receptor cytoplasmic domain into the cytosol involves two separate cleavage events. Molecular and Cellular Biology. 2023;**24**:454-464. DOI: 10.1128/MCB.24.1.454-464.2004

[8] Wen J, Liu D, Zhao L. Small molecules targeting γ-secretase and their potential biological applications. European Journal of Medicinal Chemistry. 2022;**232**:114169. DOI: 10.1016/j.ejmech.2022.114169

[9] Emoto T, Lu J, Sivasubramaniyam T, et al. Colony stimulating factor-1 producing endothelial cells and mesenchymal stromal cells maintain monocytes within a perivascular bone marrow niche. Immunity. 2022;**55**:862-878. DOI: 10.1016/j.immuni.2022.04.005

[10] Chitu V, Gökhan Ş, Stanley ER. Modeling CSF-1 receptor deficiency diseases–how close are we? FEBS Journal. 2021;**289**:5049-5073. DOI: 10.1111/febs.16085

[11] Li M, He L, Zhu J. Targeting tumor-associated macrophages for cancer treatment. Cell & Bioscience. 2022;**12**:85. DOI: 10.1186/s13578-022-00823-5

[12] Bejarano L, Jordão MJ, Joyce JA. Therapeutic targeting of the tumor microenvironment. Cancer Discovery. 2021;**11**:933-959. DOI: 10.1158/2159-8290.CD-20-1808

[13] Zhu S, Luo Z, Li X, et al. Tumor-associated macrophages: Role in tumorigenesis and immunotherapy implications. Journal of Cancer. 2021;**12**:54-64. DOI: 10.7150/jca.49692

[14] Tie Y, Tang F, Wei YQ, et al. Immunosuppressive cells in cancer: Mechanisms and potential therapeutic targets. Journal of Hematology &

Oncology. 2022;**15**:61. DOI: 10.1186/s13045-022-01282-8

[15] Duan Z, Luo Y. Targeting macrophages in cancer immunotherapy. Signal Transduction and Targeted Therapy. 2021;**6**:127. DOI: 10.1038/s41392-021-00506-6

[16] Wei J, Chen P, Gupta P, et al. Immune biology of glioma-associated macrophages and microglia: Functional and therapeutic implications. Neuro-Oncology. 2020;**22**:180-194. DOI: 10.1093/neuonc/noz212

[17] Tan IL, Arifa RDN, Rallapalli H, et al. CSF1R inhibition depletes tumor-associated macrophages and attenuates tumor progression in a mouse sonic hedgehog-medulloblastoma model. Oncogene. 2021;**40**:396-407. DOI: 10.1038/s41388-020-01536-0

[18] Yeung J, Yaghoobi V, Miyagishima D, et al. Targeting the CSF1/CSF1R axis is a potential treatment strategy for malignant meningiomas. Neuro-Oncology. 2021;**23**:1922-1935. DOI: 10.1093/neuonc/noab075

[19] Shi X, Kaller M, Rokavec M, et al. Characterization of a p53/miR-34a/CSF1R/STAT3 feedback loop in colorectal cancer. Cellular and Molecular Gastroenterology and Hepatology. 2020;**10**:391-418. DOI: 10.1016/j.jcmgh.2020.04.002

[20] Edwards DK, Watanabe-Smith K, Rofelty A, et al. CSF1R inhibitors exhibit antitumor activity in acute myeloid leukemia by blocking paracrine signals from support cells. Blood. 2019;**133**:588-599. DOI: 10.1182/blood-2018-03-838946

[21] Crotty EE, Smith S, Brasel K, et al. Medulloblastoma recurrence and metastatic spread are independent of colony-stimulating factor 1 receptor signaling and macrophage survival. Journal of Neuro-Oncology. 2021;**153**:225-237. DOI: 10.1007/s11060-021-03767-x

[22] Butowski N, Colman H, De Groot JF, et al. Orally administered colony stimulating factor 1 receptor inhibitor PLX3397 in recurrent glioblastoma: An ivy foundation early phase clinical trials consortium phase II study. Neuro-Oncology. 2015;**18**:557-564. DOI: 10.1093/neuonc/nov245

[23] Pettersen EF, Goddard TD, Huang CC, et al. UCSF chimera—A visualization system for exploratory research and analysis. Journal of Computational Chemistry. 2004;**25**:1605-1612. DOI: 10.1002/jcc.20084

[24] Ries CH, Cannarile MA, Hoves S, et al. Targeting tumor-associated macrophages with anti-CSF-1R antibody reveals a strategy for cancer therapy. Cancer Cell. 2014;**25**:846-859. DOI: 10.1016/j.ccr.2014.05.016

[25] Gelderblom H, de Sande MV. Pexidartinib: First approved systemic therapy for patients with tenosynovial giant cell tumor. Future Oncology. 2020;**16**:2345-2356. DOI: 10.2217/fon-2020-0542

[26] Wen J, Wang S, Guo R, et al. CSF1R inhibitors are emerging immunotherapeutic drugs for cancer treatment. European Journal of Medicinal Chemistry. 2023;**245**:114884. DOI: 10.1016/j.ejmech.2022.114884

[27] Zitvogel L, Rusakiewicz S, Routy B, et al. Immunological off-target effects of imatinib. Nature Reviews Clinical Oncology. 2016;**13**:431-446. DOI: 10.1038/nrclinonc.2016.41

[28] Lamb YN. Pexidartinib: First approval. Drugs. 2019;**79**:1805-1812. DOI: 10.1007/s40265-019-01210-0

[29] Andersen BM, Faust Akl C, Wheeler MA, et al. Glial and myeloid heterogeneity in the brain tumour microenvironment. Nature Review Cancer. 2021;**21**:786-802. DOI: 10.1038/s41568-021-00397-3

[30] Xu JM, Wang Y, Chen YL, et al. Sulfatinib, a novel kinase inhibitor, in patients with advanced solid tumors: Results from a phase I study. Oncotarget. 2017;**8**:42076-42086. DOI: 10.18632/oncotarget.14942

[31] Chen J, Ji Q, Wang Y, et al. The efficacy and safety of anti–PD-1 antibody toripalimab combined with surufatinib in neoadjuvant treatment of locally advanced thyroid cancer: A phase II study. Journal of Clinical Oncology. 2022;**40**:6048. DOI: 10.1200/JCO.2022.40.16_suppl.6084

[32] Caldwell TM, Ahn YM, Bulfer SL, et al. Discovery of vimseltinib (DCC-3014), a highly selective CSF1R switch-control kinase inhibitor, in clinical development for the treatment of tenosynovial giant cell tumor (TGCT). Bioorganic & Medicinal Chemistry Letter. 2022;**74**:128928. DOI: 10.1016/j.bmcl.2022.128928

[33] Rosenbaum E, Movva S, Kelly CM, et al. A phase 1b study of avelumab plus DCC-3014, a potent and selective inhibitor of colony stimulating factor 1 receptor (CSF1R), in patients with advanced high-grade sarcoma. Journal of Clinical Oncology. 2021;**39**:11549. DOI: 10.1200/JCO.2021.39.15_suppl.11549

[34] Tap WD, Wagner AJ, Sharma MG, et al. MOTION: A randomized, phase 3, placebo-controlled, double-blind study of vimseltinib (DCC-3014) for the treatment of tenosynovial giant cell tumor. Journal of Clinical Oncology. 2022;**40**:TPS11590. DOI: 10.1200/JCO.2022.40.16_suppl.TPS11590

[35] Yang S, Zhao B, Zhang M, et al. Abstract LB-288: A highly selective small molecule CSF-1R inhibitor demonstrates strong immunomodulatory activity in syngeneic models. Cancer Research. 2018;**78**:LB-288. DOI: 10.1158/1538-7445.AM2018-LB-288

[36] Falchook GS, Liang Y, Harvey RD, et al. First-in-human phase 1 study of pimicotinib (ABSK021), a CSF-1R inhibitor, in patients with advanced solid tumors. Journal of Clinical Oncology. 2023;**41**:3100. DOI: 10.1200/JCO.2023.41.16_suppl.3100

[37] Yao L, Zhou Y, Li B, et al. Efficacy and safety profile of pimicotinib (ABSK021) in tenosynovial giant cell tumor (TGCT): Phase 1b update. Journal of Clinical Oncology. 2023;**41**:11559. DOI: 10.1200/JCO.2023.41.16_suppl.11559

[38] von Tresckow B, Morschhauser F, Ribrag V, et al. An open-label, multicenter, phase I/II study of JNJ-40346527, a CSF-1R inhibitor, in patients with relapsed or refractory Hodgkin lymphoma. Clinical Cancer Research. 2015;**21**:1843-1850. DOI: 10.1158/1078-0432.CCR-14-1845

[39] Fang Y, He Y, Wu C, et al. Magnetism-mediated targeting hyperthermia-immunotherapy in "cold" tumor with CSF1R inhibitor. Theranostics. 2021;**11**:6860-6872. DOI: 10.7150/thno.57511

[40] Lin C, Gil-Martin M, Bauer TM, et al. Abstract CT171: Phase I study of BLZ945 alone and with spartalizumab (PDR001) in patients (pts) with advanced solid tumors. Cancer Research. 2020;**80**:CT171. DOI: 10.1158/1538-7445.AM2020-CT171

[41] Bendell JC, Tolcher AW, Jones SF, et al. A phase 1 study of ARRY-382, an oral inhibitor of colony-stimulating

factor-1 receptor (CSF1R), in patients with advanced or metastatic cancers. Molecular Cancer Therapy. 2013;**12**:A252. DOI: 10.1158/1535-7163.TARG-13-A252

[42] Harb WA, Johnson ML, Goldman JW, et al. A phase 1b/2 study of ARRY-382, an oral inhibitor of colony stimulating factor 1 receptor (CSF1R), in combination with pembrolizumab (Pembro) for the treatment of patients (pts) with advanced solid tumors. Journal of Clinical Oncology. 2017;**35**:TPS3110. DOI: 10.1200/JCO.2017.35.15_suppl.TPS3110

[43] Ciomei M, Zanetta L, Lussana F, et al. A phase I/II study of NMS-03592088, a FLT3, KIT and CSF1R inhibitor, in patients with relapsed or refractory AML or CMML. Blood. 2019;**134**:3855. DOI: 10.1182/blood-2019-121954

[44] Curti A, Rambaldi A, Cattaneo C, et al. Abstract CT025: NMS-03592088, a novel, potent FLT3, KIT and CSF1R inhibitor with activity in FLT3 positive acute myeloid leukemia patients with prior FLT3 inhibitor experience. Cancer Research. 2023;**83**:CT025. DOI: 10.1158/1538-7445.AM2023-CT025

[45] Yang YI, Kang H, Park D, et al. Q702, selective Axl, Mer and CSF1R triple kinase inhibitor with dual potentials leading to tumor regression: Immuno-oncology therapy and targeted cancer therapy. Cancer Research. 2019;**79**:4139. DOI: 10.1158/1538-7445.AM2019-4139

[46] Choi BJ, Devalingam D, Alistar A, et al. Abstract 2255: Patient pharmacodynamic biomarker and pk evaluation results from an ongoing phase I dose-escalation study of q702, an axl, mer and csf1r kinase inhibitor in patients with advanced solid tumors. Cancer Research. 2023;**83**:2255. DOI: 10.1158/1538-7445.AM2023-2255

[47] Deng W, Zhai D, Rogers E, et al. TPX-0022, a polypharmacology inhibitor of MET/CSF1R/SRC inhibits tumor growth by promoting anti-tumor immune responses. Cancer Research. 2019;**79**:1325. DOI: 10.1158/1538-7445.AM2019-1325

[48] Hong DS, Catenacci D, Bazhenova L, et al. Preliminary interim data of elzovantinib (TPX-0022), a novel inhibitor of MET/SRC/CSF1R, in patients with advanced solid tumors harboring genetic alterations in MET: Update from the phase 1 SHIELD-1 trial. Molecular Cancer Therapeutics. 2021;**20**:P225. DOI: 10.1158/1535-7163.TARG-21-P225

[49] Spangenberg E, Severson PL, Hohsfield LA, et al. Sustained microglial depletion with CSF1R inhibitor impairs parenchymal plaque development in an Alzheimer's disease model. Nature Communications. 2019;**10**:3758. DOI: 10.1038/s41467-019-11674-z

[50] Armstrong RC, Belli B, Rowbottom MW, et al. AC708 is a potent and selective inhibitor of CSF1R and reduces tumor associated macrophage infiltration in a breast tumor model. Cancer Research. 2013;**73**:903. DOI: 10.1158/1538-7445.AM2013-903

[51] Liu Y, Zhan Z, Kang Z, et al. Preclinical and early clinical studies of a novel compound SYHA1813 that efficiently crosses the blood-brain barrier and exhibits potent activity against glioblastoma. Acta Pharmaceutica Sinica B. 2023;**13**:4748-4764. DOI: 10.1016/j.apsb.2023.09.009

[52] Kang Z, Li S, Lin Y, et al. A phase I dose-escalation study of SYHA1813, a VEGFR and CSF1R inhibitor, in patients with recurrent high-grade gliomas or advanced solid tumors. Investigational New Drugs. 2023;**41**:296-305. DOI: 10.1007/s10637-022-01325-4

[53] Li W, Kang Z, Wu Z, et al. A phase I dose-expansion cohort of SYHA1813, a vascular endothelial growth factor receptor (VEGFR) 1-3/colony-stimulating factor 1 receptor (CSF1R) inhibitor, in patients (pts) with recurrent meningioma. Annals of Oncology. 2023;**34**:S394-S395. DOI: 10.1016/j.annonc.2023.09.1700

[54] Cruz E, Kayser V. Monoclonal antibody therapy of solid tumors: Clinical limitations and novel strategies to enhance treatment efficacy. Biologics: Targets and Therapy. 2019;**13**:33-51. DOI: 10.2147/BTT.S166310

[55] Ordentlich P. Clinical evaluation of colony-stimulating factor 1 receptor inhibitors. Seminars in Immunology. 2021;**54**:101514. DOI: 10.1016/j.smim.2021.101514

[56] Cassier PA, Italiano A, Gomez-Roca CA, et al. CSF1R inhibition with emactuzumab in locally advanced diffuse-type tenosynovial giant cell tumours of the soft tissue: A dose-escalation and dose-expansion phase 1 study. Lancet Oncology. 2015;**16**:949-956. DOI: 10.1016/S1470-2045(15)00132-1

[57] Gomez-Roca C, Cassier P, Zamarin D, et al. Anti-CSF-1R emactuzumab in combination with anti-PD-L1 atezolizumab in advanced solid tumor patients naïve or experienced for immune checkpoint blockade. Journal for Immunotherapy of Cancer. 2022;**10**:e004076. DOI: 10.1136/jitc-2021-004076

[58] Sankhala KK, Blay JY, Ganjoo KN, et al. A phase I/II dose escalation and expansion study of cabiralizumab (cabira; FPA-008), an anti-CSF1R antibody, in tenosynovial giant cell tumor (TGCT, diffuse pigmented villonodular synovitis D-PVNS). Journal of Clinical Oncology. 2017;**35**:11078. DOI: 10.1200/JCO.2017.35.15_suppl.11078

[59] Falchook GS, Peeters M, Rottey S, et al. A phase 1a/1b trial of CSF-1R inhibitor LY3022855 in combination with durvalumab or tremelimumab in patients with advanced solid tumors. Investigational New Drugs. 2021;**39**:1284-1297. DOI: 10.1007/s10637-021-01088-4

[60] Autio KA, Klebanoff CA, Schaer D, et al. Phase 1 study of LY3022855, a colony-stimulating factor-1 receptor (CSF-1R) inhibitor, in patients with metastatic breast cancer (MBC) or metastatic castration-resistant prostate cancer (MCRPC). Journal of Clinical Oncology. 2019;**37**:2548. DOI: 10.1200/JCO.2019.37.15_suppl.2548

[61] Buchbinder EI, Giobbie-Hurder A, Haq R, et al. A phase I/II study of LY3022855 with BRAF/MEK inhibition in patients with melanoma. Investigational New Drugs. 2023;**41**:551-555. DOI: 10.1007/s10637-023-01374-3

[62] Arora M, Jagasia M, Stasi AD, et al. Phase 1 study of Axatilimab (SNDX-6352), a CSF-1R humanized antibody, for chronic graft-versus-host disease after 2 or more lines of systemic treatment. Blood. 2020;**136**:722. DOI: 10.1182/blood-2020-141553

[63] Baretti M, Ding Y, Brancati M, et al. A phase II study of durvalumab (MEDI4736) in combination with a CSF-1R inhibitor (SNDX-6352) following chemotherapy or radio-embolization for patients with intrahepatic cholangiocarcinoma. Journal of Clinical Oncology. 2023;**41**:e16217. DOI: 10.1200/JCO.2023.41.16_suppl.e16217

[64] Gelderblom H, Bhadri V, Randall RL, et al. A phase 2, open-label, adaptive, dose-ranging study with

long-term extension to evaluate the safety, tolerability, efficacy, and pharmacokinetics of intra-articular AMB-05X injections in patients with tenosynovial giant cell tumor. Journal of Clinical Oncology. 2023;**41**:TPS11585. DOI: 10.1200/JCO.2023.41.16_suppl.TPS11585

[65] Papadopoulos KP, Gluck L, Martin LP, et al. First-in-human study of AMG 820, a monoclonal anti-colony-stimulating factor 1 receptor antibody, in patients with advanced solid tumors. Clinical Cancer Research. 2017;**23**:5703-5710. DOI: 10.1158/1078-0432.CCR-16-3261

[66] Gupta S, Pathak YV. Macrophage targeted delivery systems, part IV targeting macrophages for treatment of various diseases. Expert Opinion on Investigational Drugs. 2022;**31**:279-437. DOI: 10.1080/13543784.2022.2096005

[67] Callahan MK, Postow MA, Wolchok JD. Targeting T cell co-receptors for cancer therapy. Immunity. 2016;**44**:1069-1078. DOI: 10.1016/j.immuni.2016.04.023

[68] Satriano JA, Hora K, Shan Z, et al. Regulation of monocyte chemoattractant protein-1 and macrophage colony-stimulating factor-1 by IFN-gamma, tumor necrosis factor-alpha, IgG aggregates, and cAMP in mouse mesangial cells. Journal of Immunology. 1993;**150**:1971-1978. DOI: 10.4049/jimmunol.150.5.1971

[69] Neubert NJ, Schmittnaegel M, Bordry N, et al. T cell–induced CSF1 promotes melanoma resistance to PD1 blockade. Science Translational Medicine. 2018;**10**:eaan3311. DOI: 10.1126/scitranslmed.aan3311

[70] DeNardo DG, Brennan DJ, Rexhepaj E, et al. Leukocyte complexity predicts breast cancer survival and functionally regulates response to chemotherapy. Cancer Discovery. 2011;**1**:54-67. DOI: 10.1158/2159-8274.CD-10-002

[71] Olson OC, Kim H, Quail DF, et al. Tumor-associated macrophages suppress the cytotoxic activity of antimitotic agents. Cell Reports. 2017;**19**:101-113. DOI: 10.1016/j.celrep.2017.03.038

[72] Wesolowski R, Sharma N, Reebel L, et al. Phase Ib study of the combination of pexidartinib (PLX3397), a CSF-1R inhibitor, and paclitaxel in patients with advanced solid tumors. Therapeutic Advances in Medical Oncology. 2019;**11**:1758835919854238. DOI: 10.1177/1758835919854238

[73] Manji GA, Van Tine BA, Lee SM, et al. A phase I study of the combination of pexidartinib and sirolimus to target tumor-associated macrophages in unresectable sarcoma and malignant peripheral nerve sheath tumors. Clinical Cancer Research. 2021;**27**:5519-5527. DOI: 10.1158/1078-0432.CCR-21-1779

[74] Henneman L, van Miltenburg MH, Michalak EM, et al. Selective resistance to the PARP inhibitor olaparib in a mouse model for BRCA1-deficient metaplastic breast cancer. PNAS. 2015;**112**:8409-8414. DOI: 10.1073/pnas.1500223112

[75] Mehta AK, Cheney EM, Hartl CA, et al. Targeting immunosuppressive macrophages overcomes PARP inhibitor resistance in BRCA1-associated triple-negative breast cancer. Nature Cancer. 2021;**2**:66-82. DOI: 10.1038/s43018-020-00148-7

[76] Yan D, Kowal J, Akkari L, et al. Inhibition of colony stimulating factor-1 receptor abrogates microenvironment-mediated therapeutic resistance in gliomas. Oncogene. 2017;**36**:6049-6058. DOI: 10.1038/onc.2017.261

[77] Rosenbaum E, Kelly C, D'Angelo SP, et al. A phase I study of binimetinib (MEK162) combined with pexidartinib (PLX3397) in patients with advanced gastrointestinal stromal tumor. The Oncologist. 2019;**24**:1309-e983. DOI: 10.1634/theoncologist.2019-0418

[78] Pittet MJ, Michielin O, Migliorini D. Clinical relevance of tumour-associated macrophages. Nature Review Clinical Oncology. 2022;**19**:402-421. DOI: 10.1038/s41571-022-00620-6

Chapter 5

Recent Updates on Chimeric Antigen Receptor T-Cell Approaches in Cancer Immunotherapy

Maryam Sahlolbei, Amirhossein Ahmadieh-Yazdi, Mohadeseh Rostamipoor, Hamed Manoochehri, Hanie Mahaki, Hamid Tanzadehpanah, Naser Kalhor and Mohsen Sheykhhasan

Abstract

Chimeric antigen receptor (CAR) T-cell therapy is a revolutionary development in the field of cancer immunotherapy, offering a targeted approach to combat various hematologic malignancies. In this treatment, the patient's genetically modified T cells are extracted and transformed to produce chimeric antigen receptors (CARs) that are exclusive to cancer cells. These altered T cells identify, attach to, and destroy cancer cells when they are reinfused back into the patient, offering a customized course of therapy. While the CAR T-cell therapy's clinical success has been most evident in cases of acute lymphoblastic leukemia and certain types of lymphomas, ongoing research aims to extend its applicability to solid tumors. Despite its promise, challenges like cytokine release syndrome and the high cost of treatment remain. Nonetheless, CAR T-cell therapy heralds a new era in cancer treatment, offering a potentially curative approach for patients with otherwise refractory diseases.

Keywords: CAR T-cell therapy, cancer, immunotherapy, hematologic malignancies, solid tumors

1. Introduction

Cancer is a global health problem with considerable rate of mortality, so that international agency for research on cancer reported about 10 million mortality and more than 19 million new cases in 2020 [1]. Despite recent advancements in cancer therapy approaches, curing cancer remains a complex challenge. Conventional approaches such as surgery, radiotherapy and chemotherapy have limited therapeutic efficacy, underscoring the importance of developing innovative treatments [2].

Cancer cells possess the ability to escape from the immune system, leading to insufficient anti-tumor immune responses and allowing for the survival and progression of the tumor [3]. Recently, immunotherapy has become a crucial aspect of treatment for many types of diseases, notably cancer. Some immunotherapy approaches enhance the body's immunity against cancer cells, and others specifically focus on attacking tumor cells and killing them [4, 5]. Several immunotherapy techniques have been adopted in order to eradicate cancer cells, including bispecific antibodies, cytokine-induced killers (CIKs), tumor-infiltrating lymphocytes (TIL), immune checkpoint blockers, monoclonal antibodies (mAbs), tumor vaccines, and genetically engineered immune cells that express the chimeric antigen receptors (CARs) [6]. Different immune cells such as natural killer cells, macrophages, and T cells can be engineered to develop CARs to better recognize and respond against tumor cells [7]. However, lymphocyte T-based chimeric antigen receptors are still the most commonly used CARs [2]. This approach addresses the immune escapes of tumor cells, producing significantly effective T cells to target tumors [8].

CAR T cells are produced through genetic engineering of T cells derived from either the patient or a donor [9–12]. These cells are modified to express specific receptors to target a surface tumor antigen (TA) and kill cancer cells [4, 5]. Extracellular domain of CAR T cells usually is a single-chain variable fragment (scFv) followed by a hinge, a transmembrane part, and a cytosolic part that produce an intracellular signaling [13]. Unlike traditional T cells, CARs identify unprocessed antigens, along with glycolipids and structures of carbohydrates commonly found on the surface of tumor cells [14]. Also, they are completely independent of the major histocompatibility complex (MHC) [8, 15].

2. CAR T-cell therapy

Esshar's successful demonstration of genetically engineering cytotoxic T cells toward cancer cells throughout the 1980s indicated that these cells have anti-tumor potential [16]. Since that time, a new cancer treatment revolution known as chimeric antigen receptor (CAR) T-cell therapy has appeared [17].

Genetically modifying T lymphocytes to produce CAR T cells with targeted immune therapies represents a cutting-edge approach to cancer treatment [18]. This method has been used to augment the immune system's reaction against tumor cells in cases where the adaptive defenses have been ineffective [19]. Targeting tumor-associated antigens and genetically modifying T cells are two aspects of immune therapies based on CAR T cells [20]. T-cell receptors (TCR) in adaptive immunity can only recognize foreign antigens that bind to MHC. Immunotherapy based on CAR T-cells bypasses this mechanism without relying on MHC presentation and is being explored in various clinical trials for its effectiveness against different types of cancers [21]. Furthermore, this method is specific and adaptable, as the TCR domain in CAR T-cell could be modified to recognize specific antigens [22]. Additionally, treatment based on CAR T cells can form memory within patients [23].

Several solid cancers such as pancreatic, colorectal, lung, thyroid, breast, and prostate cancers, as well as hematologic malignancies like Hodgkin's and non-Hodgkin lymphomas, B-cell and T-cell lymphomas, acute myeloid leukemia (AML), acute lymphoblastic leukemia (ALL), chronic lymphocytic leukemia (CLL), and multiple myeloma (MM) have all been studied in CAR T-cell therapy [21, 24, 25]. Nevertheless, treating hematologic disorders has been one of the most prominent applications of CAR T-cell treatments.

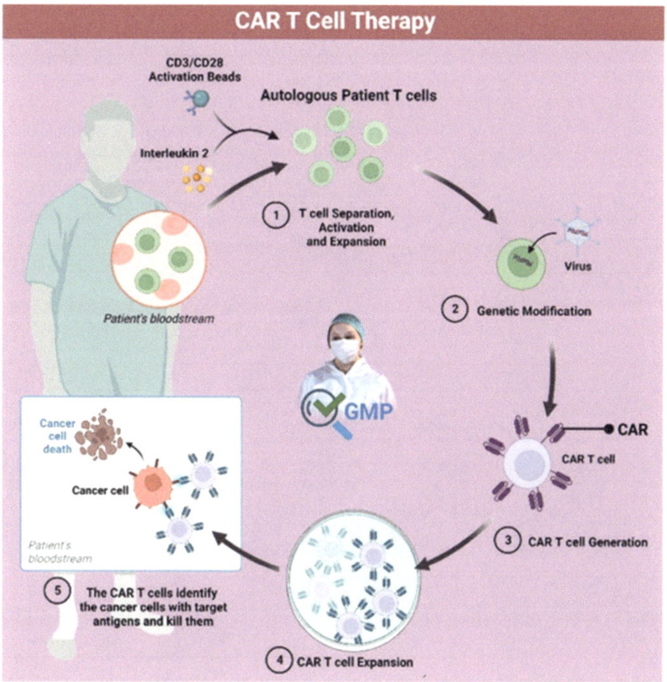

Figure 1.
The schematic chart of standard CAR T-cell production.

The Food and Drug Administration (FDA) has approved some CAR T-cell therapies to treat hematologic malignancies that express BCMA or CD19 antigens [26–28].

The standard CAR T-cell production involves five stages (**Figure 1**). Initially, T lymphocytes are extracted from patients [29]. Next, these T lymphocytes are modified with CARs, enabling them to identify tumor cells and activate themselves, thereby forming CAR T cells [8, 30]. Gene transfer methods such as viral or non-viral vectors insert CAR genes into T-lymphocyte genomes [31]. Subsequently, the modified T-lymphocyte known as CAR T-cell undergo ex vivo cultivation and stimulation through cytokines to generate a substantial quantity of CAR T lymphocytes [32]. The next phase involves reintroducing the modified T lymphocytes into the patient at the proper dosage [30]. Then, the immune system based on CAR T cells can identify and remove cancer cells that express the specific target antigen after being reinfusioned into patients [33, 34]. Finally, patients require vigilant monitoring to oversee and manage various physical responses in the subsequent days [35]. This entire process spans around 3 weeks, with CAR T-cell preparation taking approximately 2 weeks, rendering it the most time-consuming phase [23]. Both autologous and allogeneic CAR T cells have made successful transitions from preclinical to clinical stages [36]. Meanwhile, among them, autologous CAR T cells have gained approval for treating cancer patients. Over 500 treatments based on CAR T cells have been the subject of global clinical trials [37–39].

A basic CAR includes four fundamental components: an antigen-binding domain, a hinge segment, a transmembrane domain, and an intracellular domain (**Figure 2A**) [40, 41]. The antigen-binding domain is responsible for recognizing specific target antigens, while the intracellular domain delivers activation and costimulatory signals [42]. The hinge and transmembrane domains connect these two sections, also impacting their functional traits [39].

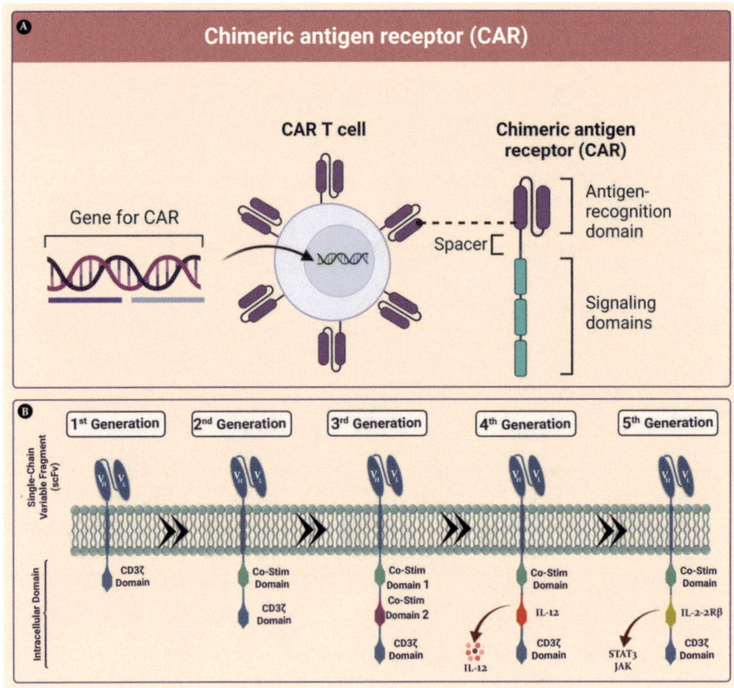

Figure 2.
The composition of distinct generations of CARs. (A) This diagram illustrates the essential elements of a CAR's extracellular, transmembrane, and intracellular domains (endodomains). (B) This diagram illustrates the progression of CAR development from the first to the fifth generation [43].

2.1 Antigen-binding domain

A CAR is a type of recombinant receptor that possesses the ability to both bind tumor antigen and stimulate T lymphocytes [44]. The antigen-binding region is the segment of the CAR T cells responsible for determining the specificity of the specific antigen [45]. The variable light chains (VL) and variable heavy chains (VH) present in antibodies (Ab) are the source of these domains [46]. These chains are connected together through a flexible connector of glycine and serine residues, creating a scFv [47]. The scFvs within CAR T cells have typically targeted tumor antigens on the extracellular surface, resulting in stimulation and growth of T cells independent of the MHC [48, 49].

The scFv has properties beyond just identifying and attaching to the target region [50]. The complementarity-determining regions' placement and the interaction between the VH and VL are two factors significantly affecting the CAR's accuracy and specificity in identifying its target [51].

The level of affinity is a crucial parameter within the antigen-binding domain, as it essentially controls the functioning of CARs [52]. The CAR's antigen-binding affinity needs to be sufficiently high for optimal performance to identify target antigens, trigger CAR T-cell signaling, and stimulate T lymphocytes [50]. Yet, it should not be excessively high to cause apoptosis by interaction with a death factor and its receptor in CAR T lymphocytes or lead to potential toxic effects [53]. While affinity is significant, it is notable that different scFvs can have different effects on CAR T-cell performance, although they have identical affinity [53]. Hence, achieving optimal CAR binding to its specific antigen necessitates consideration of additional factors, including epitope position, specific antigen density, and avoiding scFvs linked to ligand-free tonic signaling mechanisms [47].

A transmembrane domain of protein transmembrane segments such as CD3, CD8, CD28, or FcεRI fuses the scFV to the T lymphocyte [50]. This section connects to the intracellular region, which includes the intracytoplasmic regions of proteins like CD8, CD28, or CD137, as well as CD3ζ [54].

2.2 Intracellular domain

The immune receptor tyrosine-based activation motif (ITAM), usually present on the CD3ζ chain in the TCR complex and starts the costimulatory signal transduction that activates T lymphocytes, is a part of the intracellular domain [52]. An scFv that identifies recombinant tumor-associated-antigens (TAAs) and an ITAM region is created in order to manufacture CAR T cells [55]. The standard method for delivering CAR molecules into T cells is *in vitro* transfection [56]. Transfection methods can involve viral methods such as retro or lentivirus or non-viral methods like transposon and mRNA electrotransfection [54]. These components are integrated into a recombinant plasmid *in vitro* during the manufacturing process [57]. Following this, T cells are exposed to the recombinant plasmid, which makes it possible for these cells to make the receptors required for antigens on the cell membrane of tumors [55]. Post-transfection, the T lymphocytes undergo expansion. CAR T cells possess the capability to recognize and eradicate tumor cells without relying on MHC molecules, thereby overcoming potential immune evasion strategies involving reduced MHC expression by tumor cells [58]. However, the targeting is highly selective as CAR T cells can recognize tumor-specific-antigens on the cell membranes of tumor cells [59, 60]. Alongside the intracellular signaling domain, costimulatory molecules like CD137 (4-1BB) or CD28 can enhance T-lymphocyte proliferation, cytokine production, T-lymphocyte activation, and prolong *in vivo* survival [58]. These additions also boost the anti-tumor effectiveness of CART cells [61–64].

2.3 Transmembrane domain

The transmembrane domain links the intracellular and antigen-binding domains, functioning as the linker of the T-lymphocyte membrane [65]. This segment typically originates from a transmembrane receptor protein, and its selection affects the signal transduction and stimulation of the intracellular segment [48]. The transmembrane domain of CARs is likely the least understood of all their components [66]. Its main function is to attach the CAR to the membrane of the T lymphocyte [67]. However, data indicate that the transmembrane domain may be necessary for CAR T-cell function [68].

In particular, research indicates that the transmembrane domains of CAR T cells impact CAR expression levels, stability, potential signaling activity, synapse formation, and the ability to dimerize with natural signaling molecules [47, 69–71]. Numerous transmembrane domains, such as CD3ζ, CD4, CD8α, or CD28, are sourced from naturally occurring proteins [66]. As the transmembrane region is usually altered to align the requirements of the antigen-binding region or the intracellular domains, comparing the effects of different transmembrane domains on CAR function still needs to be better understood [47].

The CD3ζ transmembrane domain notably aids in CAR-mediated T-cell activation by promoting CAR dimerization and integration into native TCRs [70]. However, this advantageous effect of the CD3ζ transmembrane domain compromises the stability of CAR in comparison to those with the CD28 transmembrane domain [34]. The transmembrane domain and the hinge region seem to work together to influence CAR T-cell cytokine production as well as activation-induced cell death (AICD) [72].

Generally, research indicates that the intracellular domain with its associated transmembrane region may be the key to achieving optimum CAR T-cell signaling and activating [67]. The commonly used transmembrane domains of CD8α or CD28 may enhance CAR expression and stability [47].

2.4 An extracellular hinge or spacer domain

The hinge domain consists of members from the immunoglobulin (Ig), such as CD8, CD28, or IgG, contributing to signal transduction [73]. The antigen-binding domain extends from the transmembrane domain by extracellular segment known as the hinge or spacer domain [74]. It provides length and flexibility to cross barriers, allowing the single-chain variable fragment in the antigen-binding segment to reach the specific target antigen [75]. Crucially, due to alteration in length and composition within this area, the selected hinge seems to influence CAR functionality by changing signaling, flexibility, CAR production, epitope identification, activation strength, and epitope binding [76, 77]. Furthermore, it has been indicated that the hinge length is crucial in determining the proper intercellular spacing required to form an immune synapse [50]. The steric hindrance and the location of the specific target antigen are essential to determine the optimal hinge length [74]. While shorter spacers are better at binding epitopes distant from the membrane, longer hinges or spacers are more flexible and provide more efficient access to complex glycosylated antigens or epitopes close to the membrane [47, 78, 79]. In practical terms, the ideal spacer length is usually found through experimental methods and needs customization for each particular antigen-binding domain pairing [75]. The hinge domain frequently used the amino acid (AA) sequences found in IgG1, IgG, CD28, and CD8 [76]. However, due to potential interactions with Fcγ receptors, spacers originating from IgG may induce CAR T-lymphocyte depletion, limiting their durability *in vivo* [80]. To mitigate these effects, one can opt for an alternate hinge domain or perform further engineering of the hinge domain, considering functional or structural aspects [47].

3. CAR T-cell generations

In the lab, CAR T cells have undergone genetic modification [81]. These receptors are synthetic molecules based on TCR principles and costimulatory signaling [82]. CAR T cells are genetically engineered antibody/T-cell hybrids. The extracellular portion consists of antibody-derived heavy and light chains [83]. They are joined to form a single-stranded variable-length segment [83]. The transmembrane domain, which includes the intracellular and extracellular parts, is typically created by CD8 or IgG4 molecules [84]. The activation of T cells is mediated by an intracellular signaling domain that includes a costimulatory domain and a CD3ζ chain [85]. The intracellular domains within these structures serve as functional endpoints that trigger differentiation, cytokine production, and cytotoxic response of additional immune cells to improve the elimination of tumor cells [82]. These mechanisms enable the targeting of tumors without relying on MHC restriction [84]. Therefore, the primary focus of methods aimed at improving the effectiveness of CAR T cell therapy lies in fortifying and preserving the signaling pathways that play a crucial role in CAR T cell activation, expansion, and durability [86]. As a result, current research efforts are geared towards refining CAR structure, discovering new costimulatory molecules, and manipulating the tumor microenvironment to achieve optimal therapeutic outcomes with CAR T cells [86]. Since their introduction, the fundamental modular design of CAR T cells has not changed [86]. However, CAR T cells may be classified into five generations depending on how their intracellular signaling domain is organized (**Figure 2B**) [87].

3.1 First CAR T-cell generation

The first CARs contained only CD3 ζ-chain or an intracellular FcεRIγ domain without additional costimulatory domains [88]. The complexes were remarkably similar to the endogenous TCR but had one major limitation – they could not generate sufficient interleukin-2 (IL-2) because their response was weak, and the first-generation CARs had to be supported with exogenous IL-2 to ensure a successful response [89]. In addition, research has shown that these modified cells exhibit limited cell growth and have a short lifespan *in vivo* [90].

Following the successful integration of the CAR into the T cells, these were cultured and expanded to generate a population of CAR T cells [91]. After the patient's reinfusion, the first-generation CAR T cells identified a particular antigen in cancer cells [91]. They attached themselves to it, which led to the T-cell activation and, eventually, to the elimination of the cancer cells [92]. Nevertheless, the first-generation CAR T cells had various limitations. Their presence in the patient's body was limited, and they did not expand much, resulting in a shorter duration of response [89]. In addition, they often showed lower anti-tumor efficacy and were prone to T-cell exhaustion, leading to reduced functionality over time [92]. This has led to the need to develop the costimulatory domains further [93].

3.2 Second CAR T-cell generation

The second generation of CAR T cells aims to address the shortcomings of conventional CAR T cells, for instance, low cell proliferation, insufficient cytokine production, and short lifespan [94]. They achieve this by harnessing the power of two signals that stimulate the proliferation of T cells in the natural environment [94]. Second-generation CAR T cells have extracytoplasmic domains like CD28, 4-1BB, or OX-40 that can provide secondary signals when they encounter a tumor antigen [95]. Clinical and preclinical studies have shown that adding costimulatory signals can increase cell proliferation, cytotoxicity, and inflammatory responses by prolonging the *in vivo* half-life [96]. Further studies have also demonstrated that the composition of the costimulatory field is essential in influencing these events [96]. For example, studies have shown that 4-1BB z-CAR T cells persist in circulation more extended than CD28 z-CAR T cells [97]. On the one hand, the first factor may lead to a period of insufficient activity of CAR T cells [97]. In other words, the second factor is associated with continued activation even in the absence of antigen [98].

Treatment using second-generation CAR T cells has shown to be more successful than the first-generation CAR T cells, although it may still be linked to various side effects [50]. Cytokine release syndrome (CRS) is particularly common and has significant adverse consequence of second-generation CAR T-cell treatment [99]. The CAR T-cell activation can cause the overproduction of cytokines, leading to CRS [99, 100]. Releasing cytokines can cause a systemic inflammatory reaction, leading to symptoms similar to the flu, including fever, chills, tiredness, headache, and muscle pain [100]. In severe instances, CRS is capable of inducing high body temperature, reduced blood pressure, organ malfunctions, and potentially fatal complications [101].

Second-generation CAR T-cell treatment can cause immunological effector cell-associated neurotoxicity syndrome (ICANS), causing symptoms such as delirium, confusion, aphasia, seizures, and other neurological symptoms [102]. The cause of ICANS is believed to be caused by an immune system issue in the central nervous system; however, this is not entirely understood [103].

3.3 Third CAR T-cell generation

Third-generation CARs frameworks combine multiple costimulatory signal domains in the endodomain. Common examples of these structures are CD3ζ-CD28-OX40 or CD3ζ-CD28-41BB [104]. The CD28 costimulatory domain causes tumor cell removal, whereas the 4-1BB endodomain contributes to long-term CAR preservation [104]. However, they have been used to treat cancer with safety benefits, long-term efficacy, and increased efficacy potential [50]. However, sufficient effectiveness in contrast to second-generation CAR T cells has not yet been achieved [98, 105].

Third CAR T-cell generation therapy is founded on developing second CAR T-cell generation incorporating additional costimulatory domains [50]. Although third-generation CAR T cells aim to improve therapeutic efficacy, they may still be associated with specific side effects [6]. Third CAR T-cell generation can trigger CRS, causing systemic inflammation and flu-like symptoms like the second CAR T-cell generation [106]. The degree of side effects associated with CRS can differ from mild to very severe and threaten the patient's life [63]. Accurate monitoring and prompt management are critical to mitigate the effects of CRS [107].

Additionally, neurotoxicity from third-generation CAR T-cell treatment may result in neurological symptoms such as delirium, disorientation, seizures, and aphasia [106]. The mechanisms underlying the neurotoxicity of third-generation CAR T cells are not fully understood but are likely to be an immune-mediated response affecting the central nervous system [108]. Third-generation hematologic toxicity from third-generation CAR T-cell treatment may include a decline in platelets, RBC, and WBC [87]. These conditions can increase the risk of infections, blood complications, and the need for blood transfusions [87]. Organ damage from CAR T-cell treatment includes hepatotoxicity or liver malfunction. Monitoring liver enzymes, kidney function, and other organ parameters is essential to detect and manage toxicity [109].

3.4 Fourth-generation of TRUCK CAR T-cell

The fourth CARs are based on the second design, as multiple costimulatory domains do not enhance the effectiveness of CAR T cells [110]. The difference between these two generations is that the latter is replaced by expression cassette containing a modified protein [110]. These T cells target CAR T cells for universal cytokine-mediated killing (T cells redirected for universal cytokine-mediated killing or TRUCK), designed to deliver transgene products to cancer cells [110]. This was achieved by engineering cells to carry the nuclear factor T-cell (NFAT) response cassette that contains transgenic cytokines like IL-12 [111].

Thus, transgene expression is induced when a CD3ze-containing CAR binds to its specific target [112]. Modifying TRUCK CAR T cells requires modifying two transcriptional systems, one for CAR production and the other for inducing cytokines [112]. In preclinical models, cytokine transgene increases the effectiveness of CAR T-cell therapy in contrast to second-generation CARs [108]. The approach also managed to avoid systemic toxicity, one of the most common issues with CAR T-cell treatment [113].

TRUCK CAR T cells have been modified to produce more cytokines or immune modulators that can lead to off-target effects [113]. These side effects can include inflammation in normal tissues or unintended immune responses that can damage healthy cells and tissues [114]. Adding additional components to TRUCK CAR T cells can increase their immunogenicity, meaning the patient and the immune system recognize them as foreign [113]. This recognition can trigger an immune response against CAR T cells, reducing perseverance and effectiveness [114]. TRUCK CAR T-cell treatment can also be associated with organ toxicity, such as hepatotoxicity (liver dysfunction) or nephrotoxicity (kidney dysfunction) [114]. Monitoring organ function and managing organ toxicity are essential aspects of patient care during TRUCK CAR T-cell therapy [110].

3.5 Fifth or next-generation CAR T cells

CAR T-cell therapies have advanced rapidly in recent years to increase perseverance, proliferation, safety, and efficacy [114]. On the other hand, reducing the toxicity of off-target tumors and CAR T cells is still challenging [114]. In this regard, the new generation, which experts have already called the fifth-generation, differs from the previous and has one additional membrane receptor [114]. TRUCKS and fourth-generation CAR T cells are modified T cells activated upon exposure to their target antigen and inducing secondary transgene [110]. Subsequently, transcription happens and leads to transgene secretion into the extracellular [110]. In this approach, the hidden signal can stimulate CAR T cells, promoting their development and the formation of memory T cells [114]. Additionally, it stimulates immunological function, enhancing its response to subsequent stimulations [115]. Fifth-generation CAR T cells utilize membrane receptors and operate on a distinct principle [73]. Currently, several approaches are under testing, with the most promising one involving increased IL-2 receptors [87]. The JAK/STAT signaling cascade is facilitated by these receptors in an antigen-dependent manner [116]. One fascinating advancement in the field is the design of switch receptors [117]. Recently, there have been reports of successful coupling of drug-dependent OFF switches, resulting in CAR exhaustion, as well as ON switches, leading to activation [117]. Building upon these principles, lenalidomide-gated CARs were developed and evaluated [118]. Although these cells displayed slight effectiveness *in vitro*, they showcased improved controllability compared to earlier generations of CAR T cells [87]. Consequently, they offer a better safety profile and a more comprehensive therapeutic effect [116].

4. CAR T-cell engineering

CAR T cells, initially known as T-bodies, were first described by Yoshihisa Kuwana and his team in Japan [87]. They combined segments of antibodies with the TCR. Gideon Gross and Zelig Eshhar conceptualized the first engineered T cell with a chimeric molecule, laying the foundation for CAR T-cell therapy in Israel (in 1989) [119]. Since its inception, CAR T-cell therapy has made significant advancements during the previous several decades, evolving over five generations to reach its most advanced fifth generation. This newest generation demonstrates improved efficacy while minimizing toxicity [120]. The CAR is a receptor design made of three distinct parts [6]. These include an ectodomain, transmembrane, and intracellular domain (**Figure 2**). The ectodomain corresponds to the extracellular portion of the CAR, and it serves as the region where a hinge joins together two components [121]. CAR design has a significant impact on CAR T-cell treatment as it shows the specificity and functionality of the engineered T cells [122]. A CAR's design is made up of many essential components.

4.1 Extracellular antigen-binding domain

The extracellular domain is in control of identifying and binding itself to target antigens, which are expressed in cancer cells [52]. The scFv originates from an antibody or an alternative antigen-binding domain, such as a nanobody, and is designed to identify a particular antigen [52]. Its binding specificity determines the CAR T-cell's specificity [123]. The CAR's ability to recognize the target antigen is determined by the scFv's affinity [124]. To stimulate T cells and identify tumor cells, scFv must have a strong enough affinity [124]. A correlation that is too high can lead to AICD and potential toxicity [125]. On the other hand, poor antigen affinity makes it impossible to target healthy tissue with little antigen [126]. A recent evaluation of CARs with various affinities for scFvs that bind to related epitopes and cross-react with mouse carcinoembryonic antigen glypican 3 (GPC3) showed that high-affinity CAR T cells in the body are toxic [127]. However, low-affinity CAR T cells do not cause tissue damage while still having cytotoxic effects on antigen-positive tumor cells [127].

4.2 Hinge region

The hinge region plays a crucial role in the connection between the antigen-binding domain and the transmembrane domain of the CAR [128]. Its main purpose is to provide flexibility, enabling optimal CAR binding to the target antigen [128]. This region, also known as the spacer, is a short segment of the ectodomain derived mainly from immunoglobulin G (IgG), with occasional contributions from CD8 and CD28's hinges [87]. In addition to the antigen recognition domain, the ectodomain contains the hinge region, serving as a link between the endodomain and the ectodomain as well as the ectodomain and the TMD [87].

The primary purpose of the hinge region is to facilitate antigen attachment, enhance flexibility, and promote the formation of synapses between CAR T cells and target T cells [129]. The length of the hinge region determines the CAR's flexibility and ability to reach membrane-proximal epitopes [129]. Longer hinges provide increased flexibility and improved access to these epitopes, while shorter spacers limit flexibility and target the antigen's distal epitopes [130]. It is important to emphasize that differences in the hinge region's length may have a substantial effect on CAR antigen binding and signaling [131]. The target epitope's accessibility and location have the most effects on this [131]. While longer spacers supply more flexibility and more efficient access to membrane-proximal epitopes, shorter hinges enhance CAR T-cell activation [132]. By adding a CH2CH3 domain, for example, the distance between the T-cell surface and the CD22 epitope may be increased, boosting CD22-specific CAR activity [133]. There are substantial efforts undertaken to optimize the composition of hinges in addition to the hinge length [132]. Because of its interaction with Fcγ receptors (FcγRs), CD19-CAR built with a lengthy spacer of IgG4 hinge-CH2-CH3 has been reported to be related to a lack of *in vivo* anti-tumor efficacy [22]. However, by altering certain CH2 domain sections required for Fc receptor interaction, decreased persistence and anticancer activity may be recovered [23].

4.3 Transmembrane domain

The CAR is anchored in the T-cell membrane via the transmembrane domain [66]. This hydrophobic area stabilizes the CAR and makes sure it is positioned correctly on the surface of the T cell. The activity and stability of CAR T cells are greatly influenced by transmembrane domains, which often originate from type I proteins such as CD3, CD4, CD8α, or CD28 [70]. Interestingly, it has been shown that CARs with the CD28 transmembrane domain not only exhibit dimerization but also possess more excellent stability compared to CARs with the CD3 transmembrane region [66]. Furthermore, the transmembrane domain influences CAR expression levels directly by aiding in the removal and stabilization of the CAR inside the membrane [66, 134].

In comparing CARs with hinge and transmembrane sections made of CD28 or CD8α, recent studies have shown that the CD28 hinge can lower the antigen density cutoff needed to activate CARs [72]. Consequently, anti-CD19 CAR T cells incorporating the CD28 hinge and transmembrane regions have been found to generate more cytokine levels and exhibit increased AICD levels in contrast to CD8α hinge and transmembrane domains [72, 135]. Proline enhanced dynamic switching and local structural characteristics, such as disulfide bridges between dimeric molecules, according to further research into the biophysical and dynamic properties of CD8α, thereby enhancing signaling in a context of reduced antigen availability [72]. It is important to note that the isolated hinge domain can have a distinct function from the CAR as a whole [34]. Additionally, its interactions with the cell membrane surface might alter exchange dynamics and stabilize certain local structures [136].

4.4 Intracellular signaling domains

The CAR's intracellular signaling domains are essential for sending stimulation signals to the T cell [137]. Commonly utilized signaling domains include the CD3ζ chain of the TCR complex, which is crucial for T-cell activation [138]. Costimulatory domains such as CD28, CD134, or CD137 are employed [139]. These costimulatory domains increase T-cell activation, persistence, and proliferation, thereby improving CAR T cells' functionality and anti-tumor activity [140].

The choice and combination of intracellular signaling domains may critically impact the CAR T-cell's biological properties [138]. CARs containing only the CD3ζ signaling domain are first-generation CARs and provide essential signaling for T-cell activation [141]. Second-generation CAR T cells possess one costimulatory domain and the CD3ζ domain, while third-generation CARs incorporate two costimulatory domains [142]. Fourth-generation CAR T cells are engineered to release specific cytokines upon target antigen recognition, enhancing their anti-tumor effects [143].

CAR design also takes into account factors like the persistence of CAR T cells, resistance to immunosuppression in the microenvironment of the tumor, and avoidance of off-target toxicity [53]. Researchers are actively exploring various modifications to the CAR design to overcome these challenges and increase the overall efficacy and safety of CAR T-cell treatment [87]. These modifications involve the use of alternative spacer and hinge regions, the incorporation of inhibitory receptors to counteract immunosuppressive signaling, and switchable CARs development for more effective CAR T-cell activity regulation [144]. In summary, CAR design is crucial for CAR T-cell engineering as it controls the specificity, activation, and functionality of the engineered T cells [73]. Ongoing research and innovations in CAR design continue to advance the CAR T-cell treatment field and aim to enhance the prospect for therapy of these promising immunotherapies [145].

5. CAR T-cell evolution

The field of molecular engineering has made significant advancements, offering new avenues for addressing challenges related to CAR T-cell therapy that have emerged since its implementation in clinical settings [146]. Researchers have created innovative next-generation CAR T cells, which address the limitations of therapies using second-generation CAR T cells, such as their limited effectiveness and high toxicity [53]. These advancements aim to enhance the efficacy and safety of CAR T-cell treatment, providing promising solutions for improving patient outcomes [146].

The challenge of tumor-associated antigen escape leading to high relapse rates has spurred researchers to develop CAR T cells with dual-targeting capabilities [147]. This approach has proven successful. Clinical studies indicate that dual systems, such as CD19/BCMA for multiple myeloma and CD19/CD22 for diffuse large B-cell lymphoma, may be effective in curing these respective conditions [148]. Another promising strategy for dual-targeting involves tandem systems when a single receptor is combined with two scFv domains that bind distinct antigens [147]. Studies using preclinical models of HER2/MUC1 (breast cancer) and HER2/IL13Ra2 (glioblastoma) have shown the effectiveness of tandem CARs [149]. In all cases, compared to single-targeted CARs, dual-targeting has shown superior anti-tumor responses. Researchers have found notable variations in the responses produced by these two designs, highlighting the need to optimize and select antigens to avoid recurrence.

5.1 Dual-targeting CAR T cells

Dual-targeting CAR T-cell therapy employs a dual CAR approach to selectively target two tumor-associated antigens on specific cells [150]. Two distinct CAR T-cell structures with different antigen-binding specificities can achieve this, or a single CAR T cell can target two different antigens [150]. It is worth noting that several tumor-associated antigens are expressed in normal cells and tissues at low levels, raising concerns regarding CAR T cells' specificity in dual-targeting strategies [151]. Researchers focus on fine-tuning the antigen-binding domains to address this issue and identify specific tumor-associated post-translational modifications (PTMs) [151]. This approach aims to increase the CAR T cells' specificity, ensuring that they selectively target cancer cells while minimizing off-target effects on healthy tissues [152]. This strategy holds promise as solid tumors are recognized for their tendency to overexpress truncated O-glycans [153]. Consequently, there is ongoing investigation into using scFvs that target these modified glycans at the preclinical stage [153]. Incorporating scFvs specific to these glycans is expected to decrease the likelihood of antigen escape and reduce the toxicity of off-target effects from CAR T-cell treatments [154]. By focusing on these modified glycans, this strategy presents a viable way to raise the safety and effectiveness of CAR T-cell treatments [155].

5.2 Controlling the toxicities using switchable CAR T cells

Switchable CAR T cells offer a promising alternative to traditional CAR T therapies, addressing the challenges they present [122]. The activation of CAR T cells may be regulated, providing a completely adjustable response by using a tumor antigen-specific recombinant Fab-based 'switch' [122]. This breakthrough technology offers a solution to overcome the translational barrier faced in CAR T-cell therapy [156]. The motivation behind the development of switchable CAR T cells stems from the treatment-related toxicities often observed with conventional CAR T therapies, particularly CRS and neurotoxicity, the most common adverse effects [157]. To enhance safety, researchers have harnessed new technologies that incorporate safety switches capable of inducing apoptosis and complement-dependent cytotoxicity to deplete CAR T cells when necessary [156]. Switchable CAR T cells are created by transducing genes encoding surface antigens that can be efficiently targeted by drugs or inducible intracellular antigen effectors [87]. Once these genes are expressed, the CAR T cells become sensitive to specific drugs, enabling their depletion as required [158].

5.3 Universal CAR T-cell

The traditional CAR design is fixed, and a CAR T cell targets only one antigenic epitope [159]. This rigid design restricts the use of the drug and makes the production cost unfavorable [159]. By separating the antigen binding domain from the normal CAR's signaling domain, new CARs are created via a modular approach [160]. Therefore, the target antigen might be easily replaced or modified without the need to engineer CAR T cells [160]. Therefore, this CAR system works like a universal CAR (UniCAR) [161]. The UniCAR platform consists of a signaling module that binds to a particular epitope on the switching molecule and a switching module with an antigen-binding domain and epitope [162].

6. CAR T-cell FDA-approved

In August 2017, the United States granted its initial approval for the medical use of CAR T cells [163]. Subsequently, the FDA approved the application of CAR T cells specifically for the treatment of individuals with certain B-cell malignancies [164]. The most significant outcomes and approvals in the treatment of hematologic malignancies have been achieved through the utilization of CAR T-cell therapies targeting BCMA and CD19 [165]. The FDA has granted approval for six CAR T-cell treatments, all of which are second-generation structured, specifically for the treatment of patients with aggressive hematologic malignancies [166]. CAR T-cell treatment has shown its effectiveness in treating malignant B-cell tumors [167]. This achievement can be attributed to multiple factors, including the selected tumor cell and consistent CD19 or CD20 expression and the enhanced accessibility of CAR T cells to these targets [28]. This high rate of complete responses demonstrates CAR T-cell therapy's strong anti-tumor effects in tackling CD19-positive malignancies [168]. It demonstrates how CAR T cells may successfully remove cancer cells expressing CD19, leading to substantial clinical improvements for a significant proportion of patients [169]. The trials demonstrating the success of CAR T-cell therapy provide hope to patients with limited treatment options. The study highlights the potential of CAR T-cell therapy in combating B-cell tumors, paving the way for further research of

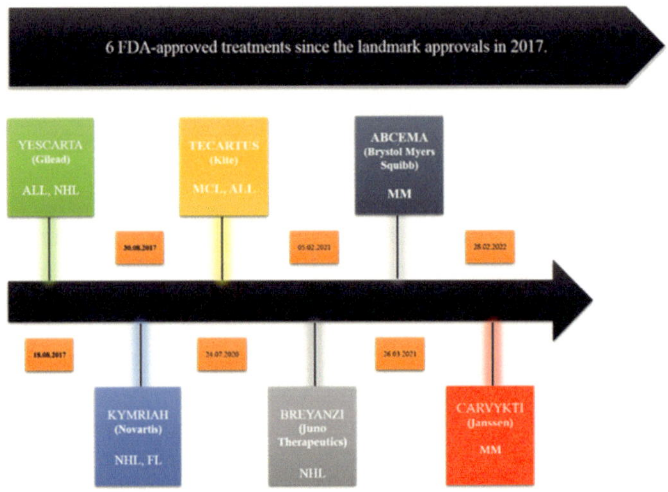

Figure 3.
Timeline of development for six CAR T-cell products authorized by the FDA in the past. A number of occasions have been identified as pivotal moments in the evolution of CAR T-cell research. Keys: ALL, acute lymphoblastic leukemia; NHL, non-Hodgkin's lymphoma; FL, follicular lymphoma; MCL, mantle cell lymphoma; MM, multiple myeloma.

CAR T-cell treatments against various cancers. **Figure 3** provides a summary of the key historical occurrences related to the advancements and developments in FDA-approved CAR T-cell product applications for cancer immunotherapy.

The FDA-approved CAR T-cell products until 2022 are listed in **Table 1**.

7. Challenges and opportunities

CAR T-cell therapy is a promising immunotherapy for certain cancer types and highlights that the research in this area is currently in a dynamic phase [8]. Due to the complexity of these biologic therapies, multiple approaches are required to provide the best possible treatment while minimizing toxicity [108]. But wider use and improved performance also face some challenges [176, 177]. Some of the main problems with CAR T-cell therapy include the following.

7.1 Cytokine release syndrome

Clinical manifestations of CRS include myalgia, hypotension, hypoxia, and fever [101]. It may produce severe fever, hemodynamic abnormalities needing vasopressor support, capillary leakage, and acute hypoxia necessitating mechanical breathing. It can also be moderate and self-limiting. Cardiovascular arrhythmias, pleural effusion, transaminitis, renal failure, coagulopathy, and hemophagocytic lymphohistiocytosis/macrophage activation syndrome (HLH/MAS) are additional clinical symptoms of CRS [51–53, 178]. The supraphysiological response of the immune system, initiated by T-cell activation and resulting in the production of various cytokines and chemokines, constitutes the fundamental pathophysiology of CRS [179]. Consensus criteria for assessing CART toxicity, including CRS, have been created lately by the American Society for Transplantation and Cellular Therapy (ASTCT) [178]. Treatment of immune cell therapy-related toxicities

DOI: http://dx.doi.org/10.5772/intechopen.1005116

Trade name/generic name	Nickname	Structure	Target antigen	Target disease	Crucial research	Approval date
Tisagenlecleucel / Kymriah™	Tisa-cel	Endodomain: CDζ-4-1BB; ectodomain: anti-CD19	CD19	Follicular lymphoma, diffuse large B-cell lymphoma, and relapsed/refractory acute lymphoblastic leukemia in children and young adults	ELIANA trial [170] JULIET trial [171]	August 2017
Axicabtagene ciloleucel/ Yescarta™	Axi-cel	Endodomain: CDζ-CD28; ectodomain: anti-CD19	CD19	Relapsed or resistant large B-cell lymphoma in adult patients	ZUMA trial [172]	October 2017
Brexucabtagene autoleucel/Tecartus™	Brexu-cel	Endodomain: CDζ-CD28; ectodomain: anti-CD19	CD19	Adult patients suffering from B-cell-ALL and relapsed/refractory MCL	ZUMA trial [173] TRANSFORM trial [51]	July 2020
Lisocabtagene maraleucel/ Breyanzi™	Liso-cel	Endodomain: CDζ-4-1BB; ectodomain: anti-CD19	CD19	Relapsed or resistant B-cell lymphoma in adult patients	TRANSFORM trial [174]	February 2021
Idecabtagene vicleucel/ Abecma™	Ide-cel	Endodomain: CDζ-4-1BB; ectodomain: anti-BCMA	BCMA	Relapsed or resistant multiple myeloma in adult patients	KarMMa trial [175]	March 2021
Ciltacabtagene autoleucel/ Carvykti™	Cilta-cel	Endodomain: CDζ-4-1BB; ectodomain: anti-BCMA	BCMA	Relapsed or resistant multiple myeloma in adult patients	CARTITUDE-trial [175]	February 2022

Abbreviations: B-cell-ALL, B-cell acute lymphoblastic leukemia, BCMA; B-cell maturation antigen; MCL, mantle cell lymphoma; MM, multiple myeloma.

Table 1.
All CAR T-cell products approved by the FDA until 2022.

requires early identification and proper management [180]. In this case, the grading system is important and has been developed since the ASTCT's current grading agreement for Adverse Events Criteria version 4.03 (CTCAE v.4.03) [100, 178].

7.2 Neurotoxicity

CAR T-cell treatment has been linked to potential neurological side effects, like ICANS [181]. Symptoms include confusion, delirium, seizures, and other neurologic abnormalities. Understanding and managing ICANS is crucial for patient safety [182]. Slow movements, tremors, lethargy, and an ataxic gait are among the usual signs of neurotoxicity [183].

CAR T-cell development is linked to high cytokine levels from immune cells, as well as increased levels of CSF and serum cytokines [99]. Therapeutic or preventive strategies that target important cytokines or preserve the integrity of the blood-brain barrier can be useful for neurotoxicity, according to cytokine profiles and autopsy investigations [184]. The consistency of neurotoxic effects linked to CAR T-cell treatment and other targeted, such as IL-2, cytotoxic chemotherapy, and blinatumomab, might be explained by this discovery [185–187].

7.3 Limited target antigens

The use of CAR T cells to treat hematologic malignancies by targeting CD19 has shown great potential [188]. On-target and off-tumor toxicities can occasionally be severe or fatal when CAR T-cell infusion is used to treat solid tumors [189]. Although both tumor and normal cells possess target antigens, not all CAR T-cell treatments exhibit appreciable off-tumor, on-target toxicities [92]. Examples of this include CAR T-cell therapies targeting carcinoembryonic antigen (CEA), mesothelin (MSLN), alpha2 (IL13Rα2), and interleukin 13 receptor [190, 191]. Moreover, preclinical trials have revealed varying levels of on-target and off-tumor toxicities among CAR T cells that target the same antigen [154]. While some toxicities were mild, others proved to be lethal, as seen in the case of fibroblast activation protein-α (FAP) targeting [192]. However, identifying appropriate target antigens for solid tumors has proven challenging [154]. Solid tumors often exhibit antigen heterogeneity, making it difficult to locate a single target capable of effectively eliminating all cancer cells [193]. CAR T cells pose a challenge in safely identifying and eliminating tumor cells due to the overexpression of targeted antigens on tumor cells [193].

7.4 Relapse and resistance

Despite initial success, some patients experience relapse or develop resistance to CAR T-cell therapy [194]. Tumor cells can evade CAR T-cell recognition by downregulating target antigens, altering antigen expression profiles, or creating other immune evasion mechanisms [24]. Overcoming resistance and preventing relapse are ongoing challenges in CAR T therapy [194]. The production of CAR T cells from leukapheresis lymphocytes, a type of patient cell, can significantly complicate drug production and potentially lead to failure [108]. In up to 10% of cases, this can occur due to either a reduction in the patient's total T-cell count or the suppression induced by their monocytes [195]. Additionally, it may result from the autologous T cells not functioning correctly in patients undergoing intense pretreatment [195]. In most cases, failure results either from the primary inability to effectively stimulate an immunological response *in vivo* or from T cells' inability to endure [196]. The mechanisms of early T-cell failure remain to be well understood [196]. Nevertheless, increasing the dose of CAR T cells cannot solve the problem, as they are only partially dose-dependent [197]. Conversely, enhancing the dose of CAR T cells may increase toxicity without increasing the efficacy of the response [123]. Combination therapies are used to stop resistance to chemotherapy or antibiotics [197]. In this approach, CAR T-cell therapy can utilize multiple antigens and immunomodulatory strategies to improve current outcomes [157]. Combining synthetic immunotherapy with checkpoint inhibitors allows for more effective treatment of recurrent and resistant B-cell malignancies, according to data from several bispecific CAR T cells evaluated in clinical studies [198]. Long-term monitoring of patients who have received CAR T therapy is necessary to understand possible relapses or secondary malignancies [157].

7.5 Manufacturing complexity

CAR T-cell production involves a complex process involving patient T-cell collection, manipulation, laboratory genetic modification, cell expansion, and infusion back into the patient [157, 199]. Standardizing and streamlining manufacturing processes is necessary to make CAR T-cell therapy more accessible and cost-effective [43]. Quality control measures are particularly important to autologous CAR T-cell therapy, as each "lot" of ingredients must be tested [43]. Timeliness is important to prevent the degradation of CAR T-cell products before infusion or cryopreservation [200]. According to the current European Union regulations, CAR T-cell therapy is classified as advanced therapy medicinal products (ATMPs) [201]. ATMPs are further categorized under EU Regulation 1394/2007, with gene therapy medical products (GTMPs) being a subset [202]. This classification includes four groups, among which CAR T cells, whether allogeneic or autologous, are encompassed, along with other treatments [202]. The Public Health Service Act (Section 351) regulates CAR T-cell therapy in the United States, requiring approval before it can be pre-marketed through conventional clinical trials [203]. The FDA and European Medicine Agency (EMA) have issued crucial guidelines for the advancement of gene and cell therapy [5].

8. Conclusion

CAR T-cell therapy is an immunotherapy that has been incredibly successful in treating certain types of cancer. Looking to the future, there are many promising and potential advances for CAR T-cell therapy:

- CAR T-cell therapy is expanding treatment options for hematologic malignancies such as leukemia and lymphoma, thereby broadening the range of cancers that can be successfully treated. The creation of CAR T-cell treatments that are successful in killing cancer cells is a current area of research focus.

- CAR T-cell therapy is a successful treatment, but it can occasionally cause serious adverse effects like neurotoxicity and CRS. Future advances to improve the safety of CAR T-cell therapy by modifying the CAR design. Given the specificity and design of CAR and virtually unlimited administration, control, and genome editing. Clinical trials are underway for CAR T-cell-based products for gene insertion, aiming to enhance tumor treatment and boost CAR T-cell production.

It will be important that these new measures capture as much information as possible from previous research. Clinical trials are underway for CAR T-cell-based products for gene insertion, aiming to enhance tumor treatment and boost CAR T-cell production.

Acknowledgements

We express our deepest gratitude to Dr. Piao Yang for her help in the Abstract preparation.

Conflict of interest

The authors declare no conflict of interest.

Acronyms and abbreviations

CAR	chimeric antigen receptor
CARs	chimeric antigen receptors
CIKs	cytokine-induced killers
TIL	tumor-infiltrating lymphocytes
mAbs	immune checkpoint blockers, monoclonal antibodies
TA	tumor antigen
scFv	single-chain variable fragments
MHC	major histocompatibility complex
TCR	T-cell receptors
AML	acute myeloid leukemia
ALL	acute lymphoblastic leukemia
CLL	chronic lymphocytic leukemia
MM	multiple myeloma
VL	variable light chains
VH	variable heavy chains
Ab	antibodies
ITAM	immune receptor tyrosine-based activation motif
TAAs	tumor-associated-antigens
AICD	activation-induced cell death
Ig	immunoglobulin
AA	amino acid
IL-2	interleukin-2
CRS	cytokine release syndrome
ICANS	immunological effector cell-associated neurotoxicity syndrome
TRUCK	T cells redirected for universal cytokine-mediated killing
NFAT	nuclear factor T-cell
GPC3	glypican 3
IgG	immunoglobulin G
FcγRs	Fcγ receptors
PTMs	post-translational modifications
ASTCT	American Society for Transplantation and Cellular Therapy
CEA	carcinoembryonic antigen
MSLN	mesothelin

IL13Rα2	alpha2
FAP	fibroblast activation protein-α
ATMPs	advanced therapy medicinal products
GTMPs	gene therapy medicinal products
EMA	European Medicine Agency

Author details

Maryam Sahlolbei[1†], Amirhossein Ahmadieh-Yazdi[2†], Mohadeseh Rostamipoor[3†], Hamed Manoochehri[3†], Hanie Mahaki[4†], Hamid Tanzadehpanah[5†], Naser Kalhor[6] and Mohsen Sheykhhasan[7*]

1 Faculty of Advanced Technologies in Medicine, Department of Molecular Medicine, Iran University of Medical Sciences, Tehran, Iran

2 Stem Cell Biology Research Center, Yazd Reproductive Sciences Institute, Shahid Sadoughi University of Medical Sciences, Yazd, Iran

3 The Persian Gulf Marine Biotechnology Research Center, The Persian Gulf Biomedical Sciences Research Institute, Bushehr University of Medical Sciences, Bushehr, Iran

4 Vascular and Endovascular Surgery Research Center, Mashhad University of Medical Sciences, Mashhad, Iran

5 Antimicrobial Resistance Research Center, Mashhad University of Medical Sciences, Mashhad, Iran

6 Department of Mesenchymal Stem Cells, Academic Center for Education, Culture and Research, Qom, Iran

7 Cellular and Molecular Research Center, Qom University of Medical Sciences, Qom, Iran

*Address all correspondence to: mohsen.sh2009@gmail.com

†These authors contributed equally.

References

[1] Bray F et al. Global cancer statistics 2018: GLOBOCAN estimates of incidence and mortality worldwide for 36 cancers in 185 countries. CA: A Cancer Journal for Clinicians. 2018;**68**(6):394-424

[2] Mehrabadi AZ et al. Therapeutic potential of CAR T cell in malignancies: A scoping review. Biomedicine & Pharmacotherapy. 2022;**146**:112512

[3] Perales MA et al. Building a safer and faster CAR: Seatbelts, airbags, and CRISPR. Biology of Blood and Marrow Transplantation. 2018;**24**(1):27-31

[4] McGuirk J et al. Building blocks for institutional preparation of CTL019 delivery. Cytotherapy. 2017;**19**(9):1015-1024

[5] Sharpe M, Mount N. Genetically modified T cells in cancer therapy: Opportunities and challenges. Disease Models & Mechanisms. 2015;**8**(4):337-350

[6] Ye B et al. Engineering chimeric antigen receptor-T cells for cancer treatment. Molecular Cancer. 2018;**17**(1):1-16

[7] Zabel M, Tauber PA, Pickl WF. The making and function of CAR cells. Immunology Letters. 2019;**212**:53-69

[8] Miliotou AN, Papadopoulou LC. CAR T-cell therapy: A new era in cancer immunotherapy. Current Pharmaceutical Biotechnology. 2018;**19**(1):5-18

[9] Sheykhhasan M, Manoochehri H, Dama P. Use of CAR T-cell for acute lymphoblastic leukemia (ALL) treatment: A review study. Cancer Gene Therapy. 2022;**29**(8-9):1080-1096

[10] Akhoundi M et al. CAR T cell therapy as a promising approach in cancer immunotherapy: Challenges and opportunities. Cellular Oncology (Dordrecht). 2021;**44**(3):495-523

[11] Mohammadi M et al. Therapeutic roles of CAR T cells in infectious diseases: Clinical lessons learnt from cancer. Reviews in Medical Virology. 2022;**32**(4):e2325

[12] Poondla N et al. The promise of CAR T-cell therapy for the treatment of cancer stem cells: A short review. Current Stem Cell Research & Therapy. 2022;**17**(5):400-406

[13] Sansom MS, Weinstein H. Hinges, swivels and switches: The role of prolines in signalling via transmembrane α-helices. Trends in Pharmacological Sciences. 2000;**21**(11):445-451

[14] Smets LA, van Beek WP. Carbohydrates of the tumor cell surface. Biochimica et Biophysica Acta (BBA)-Reviews on Cancer. 1984;**738**(4):237-249

[15] Guzman G et al. CAR-T therapies in solid tumors: Opportunities and challenges. Current Oncology Reports. 2023;**25**(5):479-489

[16] Straetemans T. Towards Clinical TCR Gene Therapy: Tumor Models and Receptors. Rotterdam: Erasmus University; 2012

[17] Gross G, Waks T, Eshhar Z. Expression of immunoglobulin-T-cell receptor chimeric molecules as functional receptors with antibody-type specificity. Proceedings of the National Academy of Sciences. 1989;**86**(24):10024-10028

[18] Ma S et al. Current progress in CAR-T cell therapy for solid tumors. International Journal of Biological Sciences. 2019;**15**(12):2548

[19] Aparicio C et al. Cell therapy for colorectal cancer: The promise of chimeric antigen receptor (CAR)-T cells. International Journal of Molecular Sciences. 2021;**22**(21):11781

[20] Tian Y et al. Gene modification strategies for next-generation CAR T cells against solid cancers. Journal of Hematology & Oncology. 2020;**13**(1):1-16

[21] Jogalekar MP et al. CAR T-cell-based gene therapy for cancers: New perspectives, challenges, and clinical developments. 2022;**13**:925985

[22] Wu L et al. Signaling from T cell receptors (TCRs) and chimeric antigen receptors (CARs) on T cells. Cellular & Molecular Immunology. 2020;**17**(6):600-612

[23] Zhao L, Cao YJ. Engineered T cell therapy for cancer in the clinic. 2019;**10**:2250

[24] Qu C et al. Tumor buster-where will the CAR-T cell therapy 'missile' go? Molecular Cancer. 2022;**21**(1):201

[25] Chohan KL, Siegler EL, Kenderian SS. CAR-T cell therapy: The efficacy and toxicity balance. Current Hematologic Malignancy Reports. 2023;**18**(2):9-18

[26] Gumber D, Wang LD. Improving CAR-T immunotherapy: Overcoming the challenges of T cell exhaustion. EBioMedicine. 2022;**77**

[27] Selli ME et al. Costimulatory domains direct distinct fates of CAR-driven T-cell dysfunction. Blood. 2023;**141**(26):3153-3165

[28] Tong C et al. Optimized tandem CD19/CD20 CAR-engineered T cells in refractory/relapsed B-cell lymphoma. Blood, The Journal of the American Society of Hematology. 2020;**136**(14):1632-1644

[29] Demaret J et al. Monitoring CAR T-cells using flow cytometry. Cytometry Part B: Clinical Cytometry. 2021;**100**(2):218-224

[30] Lin Y et al. Idecabtagene vicleucel (ide-cel, bb2121), a BCMA-directed CAR T cell therapy, in patients with relapsed and refractory multiple myeloma: Updated results from phase 1 CRB-401 study. Blood. 2020;**136**:26-27

[31] Harris E. Optimizing Non-Viral Gene Delivery to T Lymphocytes for CAR-T Cell Therapy. Master's Thesis. Villanova University; 2020

[32] Xu Y et al. Closely related T-memory stem cells correlate with in vivo expansion of CAR. CD19-T cells and are preserved by IL-7 and IL-15. Blood, The Journal of the American Society of Hematology. 2014;**123**(24):3750-3759

[33] Sadelain M, Brentjens R, Rivière I. The basic principles of chimeric antigen receptor design. 2013;**3**(4):388-398

[34] Dotti G et al. Design and development of therapies using chimeric antigen receptor-expressing T cells. Immunological Reviews. 2014;**257**(1):107-126

[35] Perica K et al. Adoptive T cell immunotherapy for cancer. Rambam Maimonides Medical Journal. 2015;**6**:1

[36] Cheadle EJ et al. CAR T cells: Driving the road from the laboratory to the clinic. Immunological Reviews. 2014;**257**(1):91-106

[37] Papathanasiou MM et al. Autologous CAR T-cell therapies supply chain: Challenges and opportunities? Cancer Gene Therapy. 2020;**27**(10-11):799-809

[38] Depil S et al. 'Off-the-shelf' allogeneic CAR T cells: Development and challenges. Nature Reviews Drug Discovery. 2020;**19**(3):185-199

[39] Khan AN et al. Immunogenicity of CAR-T cell therapeutics: Evidence, mechanism and mitigation. Frontiers in Immunology. 2022;**13**:886546

[40] López-Gómez M et al. Cancer in developing countries: The next most preventable pandemic. The Global Problem of Cancer. 2013;**88**(1):117-122

[41] Benmebarek M-R et al. Killing mechanisms of chimeric antigen receptor (CAR) T cells. International Journal of Molecular Sciences. 2019;**20**(6):1283

[42] Song J et al. Intracellular signals of T cell costimulation. Cellular & Molecular Immunology. 2008;**5**(4):239-247

[43] Sheykhhasan M et al. CAR T therapies in multiple myeloma: Unleashing the future. Cancer Gene Therapy. 2024. DOI: 10.1038/s41417-024-00750-2

[44] Ramos CA, Dotti G. Chimeric antigen receptor (CAR)-engineered lymphocytes for cancer therapy. Expert Opinion on Biological Therapy. 2011;**11**(7):855-873

[45] Hanssens H et al. The antigen-binding moiety in the driver's seat of CARs. Medicinal Research Reviews. 2022;**42**(1):306-342

[46] Sun Z et al. Construction of a large size human immunoglobulin heavy chain variable (VH) domain library, isolation and characterization of novel human antibody VH domains targeting PD-L1 and CD22. Frontiers in Immunology. 2022;**13**:869825

[47] Sterner RC, Sterner RM. CAR-T cell therapy: Current limitations and potential strategies. Blood Cancer Journal. 2021;**11**(4):69

[48] Maude SL et al. Tisagenlecleucel in children and young adults with B-cell lymphoblastic leukemia. New England Journal of Medicine. 2018;**378**(5):439-448

[49] Kenderian SS et al. Chimeric antigen receptor T cells and hematopoietic cell transplantation: How not to put the CART before the horse. Biology of Blood and Marrow Transplantation. 2017;**23**(2):235-246

[50] Srivastava S, Riddell SR. Engineering CAR-T cells: Design concepts. Trends in Immunology. 2015;**36**(8):494-502

[51] Lu J, Jiang GJMC. The journey of CAR-T therapy in hematological malignancies. Molecular Cancer. 2022;**21**(1):1-15

[52] Wu Y, Jiang S, Ying T. From therapeutic antibodies to chimeric antigen receptors (CARs): Making better CARs based on antigen-binding domain. Expert Opinion on Biological Therapy. 2016;**16**(12):1469-1478

[53] Brudno JN, Kochenderfer JN. Toxicities of chimeric antigen receptor T cells: Recognition and management. Blood, The Journal of the American Society of Hematology. 2016;**127**(26):3321-3330

[54] Schepisi G et al. CAR-T cell therapy: A potential new strategy against prostate cancer. Journal for Immunotherapy of Cancer. 2019;**7**:1-11

[55] Giordano Attianese GMP, Ash S, Irving M. Coengineering specificity, safety, and function into T cells for cancer immunotherapy. Immunological Reviews. 2023;**320**(1):166-198

[56] Kumar AR et al. Materials for improving immune cell transfection. Advanced Materials. 2021;**33**(21):2007421

[57] Poorebrahim M et al. Production of CAR T-cells by GMP-grade lentiviral vectors: Latest advances and future prospects. Critical Reviews in Clinical Laboratory Sciences. 2019;**56**(6):393-419

[58] Martinez M, Moon EK. CAR T cells for solid tumors: New strategies for finding, infiltrating, and surviving in the tumor microenvironment. Frontiers in Immunology. 2019;**10**:128

[59] Zhang Q et al. CAR-T cell therapy in cancer: Tribulations and road ahead. Journal of Immunology Research. 2020;**2020**

[60] Pajarinen J et al. Mesenchymal stem cell-macrophage crosstalk and bone healing. Biomaterials. 2019;**196**:80-89

[61] Neelapu SS et al. Axicabtagene ciloleucel CAR T-cell therapy in refractory large B-cell lymphoma. New England Journal of Medicine. 2017;**377**(26):2531-2544

[62] Mullard A. FDA approves first CAR T therapy. InsideHealthPolicy.com's FDA Week. 2017;**16**(10):669-670

[63] Kalos M et al. T cells with chimeric antigen receptors have potent antitumor effects and can establish memory in patients with advanced leukemia. Science Translational Medicine. 2011;**3**(95):95ra73-95ra73

[64] Wang Z et al. Current status and perspectives of chimeric antigen receptor modified T cells for cancer treatment. Protein & Cell. 2017;**8**(12):896-925

[65] Bentley GA, Mariuzza RA. The structure of the T cell antigen receptor. Annual Review of Immunology. 1996;**14**(1):563-590

[66] Fujiwara K et al. Hinge and transmembrane domains of chimeric antigen receptor regulate receptor expression and signaling threshold. Cells. 2020;**9**(5):1182

[67] Jayaraman J et al. CAR-T design: Elements and their synergistic function. eBioMedicine. 2020;**58**:102931

[68] Guedan S et al. Enhancing CAR T cell persistence through ICOS and 4-1BB costimulation. JCI Insight. 2018;**3**(1):e96976

[69] Zhang T, Wu M-R, Sentman CL. An NKp30-based chimeric antigen receptor promotes T cell effector functions and antitumor efficacy in vivo. The Journal of Immunology. 2012;**189**(5):2290-2299

[70] Bridgeman JS et al. The optimal antigen response of chimeric antigen receptors harboring the CD3ζ transmembrane domain is dependent upon incorporation of the receptor into the endogenous TCR/CD3 complex. The Journal of Immunology. 2010;**184**(12):6938-6949

[71] Sauer T et al. CD70-specific CAR T cells have potent activity against acute myeloid leukemia without HSC toxicity. Blood. 2021;**138**(4):318-330

[72] Alabanza L et al. Function of novel anti-CD19 chimeric antigen receptors with human variable regions is affected by hinge and transmembrane domains. Molecular Therapy. 2017;**25**(11):2452-2465

[73] Sadelain M, Rivière I, Riddell SJN. Therapeutic T cell engineering. Nature. 2017;**545**(7655):423-431

[74] Litman GW, Anderson MK, Rast JP. Evolution of antigen binding receptors. Annual Review of Immunology. 1999;**17**(1):109-147

[75] Mazinani M, Rahbarizadeh F. CAR-T cell potency: From structural elements to vector backbone components. Biomarker Research. 2022;**10**(1):1-24

[76] Hudecek M et al. The nonsignaling extracellular spacer domain of chimeric antigen receptors is decisive for in vivo antitumor activity. Cancer Immunology Research. 2015;**3**(2):125-135

[77] Jensen MC, Riddell SR. Designing chimeric antigen receptors to effectively and safely target tumors. Current Opinion in Immunology. 2015;**33**:9-15

[78] Guest RD et al. The role of extracellular spacer regions in the optimal design of chimeric immune receptors: Evaluation of four different scFvs and antigens. Journal of Immunotherapy. 2005;**28**(3):203-211

[79] Zah E et al. T cells expressing CD19/CD20 bi-specific chimeric antigen receptors prevent antigen escape by malignant B cells. Cancer Immunology Research. 2016;**4**(6):498-508

[80] Almåsbak H et al. Inclusion of an IgG1-Fc spacer abrogates efficacy of CD19 CAR T cells in a xenograft mouse model. Gene Therapy. 2015;**22**(5):391-403

[81] Jensen MC, Riddell SR. Design and implementation of adoptive therapy with chimeric antigen receptor-modified T cells. Immunological Reviews. 2014;**257**(1):127-144

[82] Germain RN, Stefanová I. The dynamics of T cell receptor signaling: Complex orchestration and the key roles of tempo and cooperation. Annual Review of Immunology. 1999;**17**(1):467-522

[83] Pircher M, Schirrmann T, Petrausch U. T cell engineering. Immuno-Oncology. 2015;**42**:110-135

[84] Scarfò I, Maus MV. Current approaches to increase CAR T cell potency in solid tumors: Targeting the tumor microenvironment. Journal for Immunotherapy of Cancer. 2017;**5**(1):1-8

[85] Zhang C et al. Engineering CAR-T cells. Biomarker Research. 2017;**5**(1):22

[86] Kyte JA. Strategies for improving the efficacy of CAR T cells in solid cancers. Cancers. 2022;**14**(3):571

[87] Asmamaw Dejenie T et al. Current updates on generations, approvals, and clinical trials of CAR T-cell therapy. Human Vaccines & Immunotherapeutics. 2022;**18**(6):2114254

[88] Huang R et al. Recent advances in CAR-T cell engineering. Journal of Hematology & Oncology. 2020;**13**(1):1-19

[89] Rosado-Sanchez I et al. Integration of exogenous and endogenous co-stimulatory signals by CAR-Tregs. bioRxiv. 2022. DOI: 10.11012022.11.10.516049

[90] Eshhar Z et al. Specific activation and targeting of cytotoxic lymphocytes through chimeric single chains consisting of antibody-binding domains and the gamma or zeta subunits of the immunoglobulin and T-cell receptors. Proceedings of the National Academy of Sciences of the United States of America. 1993;**90**(2):720-724

[91] Agarwal S et al. In vivo generation of CAR T cells selectively in human CD4+ lymphocytes. Molecular Therapy. 2020;**28**(8):1783-1794

[92] Levine B. Performance-enhancing drugs: Design and production of

redirected chimeric antigen receptor (CAR) T cells. Cancer Gene Therapy. 2015;**22**(2):79-84

[93] Smith AJ et al. Chimeric antigen receptor (CAR) T cell therapy for malignant cancers: Summary and perspective. Journal of Cellular Immunotherapy. 2016;**2**(2):59-68

[94] Abate-Daga D, Davila ML. CAR models: Next-generation CAR modifications for enhanced T-cell function. Molecular Therapy-Oncolytics. 2016;**3**:16014

[95] Imai C et al. Chimeric receptors with 4-1BB signaling capacity provoke potent cytotoxicity against acute lymphoblastic leukemia. Leukemia. 2004;**18**(4):676-684

[96] Qiao J, Fu Y-X. Cytokines that target immune killer cells against tumors. Cellular & Molecular Immunology. 2020;**17**(7):722-727

[97] Dwivedi A et al. Lymphocytes in cellular therapy: Functional regulation of CAR T cells. Frontiers in Immunology. 2019;**9**:3180

[98] Ramos CA et al. In vivo fate and activity of second- versus third-generation CD19-specific CAR-T cells in B cell non-Hodgkin's lymphomas. Molecular Therapy. 2018;**26**(12):2727-2737

[99] Gust J et al. Cytokines in CAR T cell–associated neurotoxicity. Frontiers in Immunology. 2020;**11**:577027

[100] Murthy H et al. Cytokine release syndrome: Current perspectives. Immuno Targets and Therapy. 2019;**8**(null):43-52

[101] Cobb DA, Lee DW. Cytokine release syndrome biology and management. The Cancer Journal. 2021;**27**(2):119-125

[102] Rice J et al. Chimeric antigen receptor T cell-related neurotoxicity: Mechanisms, clinical presentation, and approach to treatment. Current Treatment Options in Neurology. 2019;**21**:1-14

[103] Sterner RC, Sterner RM. Immune effector cell associated neurotoxicity syndrome in chimeric antigen receptor-T cell therapy. Frontiers in Immunology. 2022;**23**(1):112-121

[104] Zhang C et al. Engineering car-t cells. Biomarker Research. 2017;**5**(1):1-6

[105] Hombach AA, Rappl G, Abken H. Arming cytokine-induced killer cells with chimeric antigen receptors: CD28 outperforms combined CD28-OX40 "super-stimulation". Molecular Therapy. 2013;**21**(12):2268-2277

[106] Acharya UH et al. Management of cytokine release syndrome and neurotoxicity in chimeric antigen receptor (CAR) T cell therapy. Expert Review of Hematology. 2019;**12**(3):195-205

[107] Li Y et al. The pathogenesis, diagnosis, prevention, and treatment of CAR-T cell therapy-related adverse reactions. Frontiers in Pharmacology. 2022;**13**:950923

[108] Sathish JG et al. Challenges and approaches for the development of safer immunomodulatory biologics. Nature Reviews Drug Discovery. 2013;**12**(4):306-324

[109] Rejeski K et al. CAR-HEMATOTOX: A model for CAR T-cell-related hematologic toxicity in relapsed/refractory large B-cell lymphoma. Blood. 2021;**138**(24):2499-2513

[110] Chmielewski M, Abken H. TRUCKs: The fourth generation of CARs. Expert

Opinion on Biological Therapy. 2015;**15**(8):1145-1154

[111] Duan D et al. The BCMA-targeted fourth-generation CAR-T cells secreting IL-7 and CCL19 for therapy of refractory/recurrent multiple myeloma. Frontiers in Immunology. 2021;**12**:609421

[112] Tang L et al. Arming CAR-T cells with cytokines and more: Innovations in the fourth-generation CAR-T development. Molecular Therapy. 2023;**31**(11):3146-3162

[113] Chmielewski M, Abken H. TRUCKS, the fourth-generation CAR T cells: Current developments and clinical translation. Advances in Cell and Gene Therapy. 2020;**3**(3):e84

[114] Yi D et al. Next-generation chimeric antigen receptor T cells. Hematology/ Oncology and Stem Cell Therapy. 2022;**15**(3):11

[115] Tokarew N et al. Teaching an old dog new tricks: Next-generation CAR T cells. British Journal of Cancer. 2019;**120**(1):26-37

[116] Kagoya Y et al. A novel chimeric antigen receptor containing a JAK–STAT signaling domain mediates superior antitumor effects. Nature Medicine. 2018;**24**(3):352-359

[117] Liu X et al. A chimeric switch-receptor targeting PD1 augments the efficacy of second-generation CAR T cells in advanced solid tumors. Cancer Research. 2016;**76**(6):1578-1590

[118] Jan M et al. Reversible ON-and OFF-switch chimeric antigen receptors controlled by lenalidomide. Science Translational Medicine. 2021;**13**(575):eabb6295

[119] Bourbon E, Ghesquières H, Bachy E. CAR-T cells, from principle to clinical applications. Bulletin du Cancer. 2021;**108**(10s):S4-s17

[120] Beck A et al. Strategies and challenges for the next generation of antibody–drug conjugates. Nature Reviews Drug Discovery. 2017;**16**(5):315-337

[121] Zheng Z et al. Fine-tuning through generations: Advances in structure and production of CAR-T therapy. Cancers. 2023;**15**(13):3476

[122] Andrea AE et al. Engineering next-generation CAR-T cells for better toxicity management. International Journal of Molecular Sciences. 2020;**21**(22):8620

[123] Gardner RA et al. Intent-to-treat leukemia remission by CD19 CAR T cells of defined formulation and dose in children and young adults. Blood, The Journal of the American Society of Hematology. 2017;**129**(25):3322-3331

[124] Duan Y et al. Tuning the ignition of CAR: Optimizing the affinity of scFv to improve CAR-T therapy. Cellular and Molecular Life Sciences. 2022;**79**(1):14

[125] Künkele A et al. Functional tuning of CARs reveals signaling threshold above which CD8+ CTL antitumor potency is attenuated due to cell Fas–FasL-dependent AICD. Cancer Immunology Research. 2015;**3**(4):368-379

[126] Strohl WR, Naso M. Bispecific T-cell redirection versus chimeric antigen receptor (CAR)-T cells as approaches to kill cancer cells. Antibodies. 2019;**8**(3):41

[127] Torchia MLG et al. Rational design of chimeric antigen receptor T cells against glypican 3 decouples toxicity from therapeutic efficacy. Cytotherapy. 2022;**24**(7):720-732

[128] Wu H et al. A CH2CH3 hinge region enhances the cytotoxicity of anti-CD5 CAR-T cells targeting T cell acute lymphoblastic leukemia. International Immunopharmacology. 2023;**124**:110904

[129] Zhang A et al. Reducing hinge flexibility of CAR-T cells prolongs survival in vivo with low cytokines release. Frontiers in Immunology. 2021;**12**:724211

[130] Ahmad U et al. Chimeric antigen receptor T cell structure, its manufacturing, and related toxicities; A comprehensive review. Advances in Cancer Biology - Metastasis. 2022;**4**:100035

[131] Hirobe S et al. The effects of chimeric antigen receptor (CAR) hinge domain post-translational modifications on CAR-T cell activity. International Journal of Molecular Sciences. 2022;**23**(7):4056

[132] Qin L et al. Incorporation of a hinge domain improves the expansion of chimeric antigen receptor T cells. Journal of Hematology & Oncology. 2017;**10**:1-11

[133] Hudecek M et al. Receptor affinity and extracellular domain modifications affect tumor recognition by ROR1-specific chimeric antigen receptor T cells. Clinical Cancer Research. 2013;**19**(12):3153-3164

[134] Muller YD et al. The CD28-transmembrane domain mediates chimeric antigen receptor heterodimerization with CD28. Frontiers in Immunology. 2021;**12**:500

[135] Chen X et al. The CD8α hinge is intrinsically disordered with a dynamic exchange that includes proline cis-trans isomerization. Journal of Magnetic Resonance. 2022;**340**:107234

[136] Leick MB et al. Non-cleavable hinge enhances avidity and expansion of CAR-T cells for acute myeloid leukemia. Cancer Cell. 2022;**40**(5):494-508 e5

[137] Butler SE et al. Toward high-throughput engineering techniques for improving CAR intracellular signaling domains. Frontiers in Bioengineering and Biotechnology. 2023;**11**:1101122

[138] Karlsson H et al. Evaluation of intracellular signaling downstream chimeric antigen receptors. PLoS One. 2015;**10**(12):e0144787

[139] He Y et al. The implementation of TNFRSF co-stimulatory domains in CAR-T cells for optimal functional activity. Cancers. 2022;**14**(2):299

[140] Taraban VY et al. Expression and costimulatory effects of the TNF receptor superfamily members CD134 (OX40) and CD137 (4-1BB), and their role in the generation of anti-tumor immune responses. European Journal of Immunology. 2002;**32**(12):3617-3627

[141] Fujiwara K et al. Structure of the signal transduction domain in second-generation CAR regulates the input efficiency of CAR signals. International Journal of Molecular Sciences. 2021;**22**(5):2476

[142] Honikel MM, Olejniczak SH. Co-stimulatory receptor signaling in CAR-T cells. Biomolecules. 2022;**12**(9):1303

[143] Glienke W et al. GMP-compliant manufacturing of TRUCKs: CAR T cells targeting GD2 and releasing inducible IL-18. Frontiers in Immunology. 2022;**13**:839783

[144] Głowacki P, Rieske P. Application and design of switches used in CAR. Cells. 2022;**11**(12):1910

[145] Ahmed MME. CAR-T cell therapy: Current advances and future research

possibilities. Journal of Scientific Research in Medical and Biological Sciences. 2021;**2**(2):86-116

[146] Lee Y-H, Kim CH. Evolution of chimeric antigen receptor (CAR) T cell therapy: Current status and future perspectives. Archives of Pharmacal Research. 2019;**42**:607-616

[147] Spiegel JY et al. CAR T cells with dual targeting of CD19 and CD22 in adult patients with recurrent or refractory B cell malignancies: A phase 1 trial. Nature Medicine. 2021;**27**(8):1419-1431

[148] Guo Z et al. Preclinical and clinical advances in dual-target chimeric antigen receptor therapy for hematological malignancies. Cancer Science. 2021;**112**(4):1357-1368

[149] Du S et al. Adoptive cell therapy for cancer treatment. In: Exploration. Vol. 3, No. 4. Wiley Online Library; 2023. p. 20210058

[150] Hirabayashi K et al. Dual-targeting CAR-T cells with optimal co-stimulation and metabolic fitness enhance antitumor activity and prevent escape in solid tumors. Nature Cancer. 2021;**2**(9):904-918

[151] Larson RC et al. Anti-TACI single and dual-targeting CAR T cells overcome BCMA antigen loss in multiple myeloma. Nature Communications. 2023;**14**(1):7509

[152] Van der Schans JJ, Van de Donk NW, Mutis T. Dual targeting to overcome current challenges in multiple myeloma CAR T-cell treatment. Frontiers in Oncology. 2020;**10**:534747

[153] Raglow Z et al. Targeting glycans for CAR therapy: The advent of sweet CARs. Molecular Therapy. 2022;**30**(9):2881-2890

[154] Flugel CL et al. Overcoming on-target, off-tumour toxicity of CAR T cell therapy for solid tumours. Nature Reviews Clinical Oncology. 2023;**20**(1):49-62

[155] Xie B et al. Current status and perspectives of dual-targeting chimeric antigen receptor T-cell therapy for the treatment of Hematological malignancies. Cancers. 2022;**14**(13):3230

[156] Xin T et al. In-vivo induced CAR-T cell for the potential breakthrough to overcome the barriers of current CAR-T cell therapy. Frontiers in Oncology. 2022;**12**:809754

[157] Rafiq S, Hackett CS, Brentjens RJ. Engineering strategies to overcome the current roadblocks in CAR T cell therapy. Nature Reviews. Clinical Oncology. 2020;**17**(3):147-167

[158] Moghanloo E et al. Remote controlling of CAR-T cells and toxicity management: Molecular switches and next generation CARs. Translational Oncology. 2021;**14**(6):101070

[159] Zhao J et al. Universal CARs, universal T cells, and universal CAR T cells. Journal of Hematology & Oncology. 2018;**11**:1-9

[160] Lin H et al. Advances in universal CAR-T cell therapy. Frontiers in Immunology. 2021;**12**:744823

[161] Wermke M et al. Proof of concept for a rapidly switchable universal CAR-T platform with UniCAR-T-CD123 in relapsed/refractory AML. Blood, The Journal of the American Society of Hematology. 2021;**137**(22):3145-3148

[162] Liu D, Zhao J, Song Y. Engineering switchable and programmable universal CARs for CAR T therapy. Journal of Hematology & Oncology. 2019;**12**:1-9

[163] Braendstrup P, Levine BL, Ruella M. The long road to the first FDA-approved gene therapy: Chimeric antigen receptor T cells targeting CD19. Cytotherapy. 2020;**22**(2):57-69

[164] Demko S et al. FDA drug approval summary: Alemtuzumab as single-agent treatment for B-cell chronic lymphocytic leukemia. The Oncologist. 2008;**13**(2):167-174

[165] D'Agostino M, Raje N. Anti-BCMA CAR T-cell therapy in multiple myeloma: Can we do better? Leukemia. 2020;**34**(1):21-34

[166] DeFrancesco L. CAR-T's forge ahead, despite Juno deaths. Nature Biotechnology. 2017;**35**(1):6-8

[167] Zhang T et al. Efficiency of CD19 chimeric antigen receptor-modified T cells for treatment of B cell malignancies in phase I clinical trials: A meta-analysis. Oncotarget. 2015;**6**(32):33961

[168] Bouziana S, Bouzianas D. Anti-CD19 CAR-T cells: Digging in the dark side of the golden therapy. Critical Reviews in Oncology/Hematology. 2021;**157**:103096

[169] Hartmann J et al. Clinical development of CAR T cells—Challenges and opportunities in translating innovative treatment concepts. EMBO Molecular Medicine. 2017;**9**(9):1183-1197

[170] Thudium Mueller K et al. Tisagenlecleucel immunogenicity in relapsed/refractory acute lymphoblastic leukemia and diffuse large B-cell lymphoma. Blood Advances. 2021;**5**(23):4980-4991

[171] Maziarz RT et al. Grading of neurological toxicity in patients treated with tisagenlecleucel in the JULIET trial. Blood Advances. 2020;**4**(7):1440-1447

[172] Locke FL et al. Long-term safety and activity of axicabtagene ciloleucel in refractory large B-cell lymphoma (ZUMA-1): A single-arm, multicentre, phase 1-2 trial. The Lancet Oncology. 2019;**20**(1):31-42

[173] Lovell A. Brexucabtagene Autoleucel (Tecartus™). Oncology Times. 2022;**44**(16):10

[174] Johnson V. New data supports Breyanzi's expansion to chronic lymphocytic Leukemia. Victoria. 2023

[175] Harousseau JL. CAR-T cell therapy in myeloma: Hopes and hurdles. Blood Science. 2023;**5**(2):136

[176] Chicaybam L et al. Overhauling CAR T cells to improve efficacy, safety and cost. Cancers. 2020;**12**(9):2360

[177] Brudno JN, Kochenderfer JN. Recent advances in CAR T-cell toxicity: Mechanisms, manifestations and management. Blood Reviews. 2019;**34**:45-55

[178] Lee DW et al. ASTCT consensus grading for cytokine release syndrome and neurologic toxicity associated with immune effector cells. Biology of Blood and Marrow Transplantation. 2019;**25**(4):625-638

[179] Khadka RH et al. Management of cytokine release syndrome: An update on emerging antigen-specific T cell engaging immunotherapies. Immunotherapy. 2019;**11**(10):851-857

[180] Neelapu SS. Managing the toxicities of car T-cell therapy. Hematological Oncology. 2019;**37**:48-52

[181] Neill L, Rees J, Roddie C. Neurotoxicity—CAR T-cell therapy: What the neurologist needs to know. Practical Neurology. 2020;**20**(4):285-293

[182] Holtzman NG et al. Immune effector cell–associated neurotoxicity syndrome after chimeric antigen receptor T-cell therapy for lymphoma: Predictive biomarkers and clinical outcomes. Neuro-Oncology. 2021;**23**(1):112-121

[183] Hunter BD, Jacobson CA. CAR T-cell associated neurotoxicity: Mechanisms, clinicopathologic correlates, and future directions. JNCI: Journal of the National Cancer Institute. 2019;**111**(7):646-654

[184] Gust J et al. Endothelial activation and blood–brain barrier disruption in neurotoxicity after adoptive immunotherapy with CD19 CAR-T cells. Cancer Discovery. 2017;**7**(12):1404-1419

[185] Torre M et al. Neuropathology of a case with fatal CAR T-cell-associated cerebral edema. Journal of Neuropathology & Experimental Neurology. 2018;**77**(10):877-882

[186] Wardill HR et al. Cytokine-mediated blood brain barrier disruption as a conduit for cancer/chemotherapy-associated neurotoxicity and cognitive dysfunction. International Journal of Cancer. 2016;**139**(12):2635-2645

[187] Dutcher J et al. Kidney cancer: The cytokine working group experience (1986-2001) part II: Management of IL-2 toxicity and studies with other cytokines. Medical Oncology. 2001;**18**:209-219

[188] Zhang Y et al. An analytical biomarker for treatment of patients with recurrent B-ALL after remission induced by infusion of anti-CD19 chimeric antigen receptor T (CAR-T) cells. Science China Life Sciences. 2016;**59**:379-385

[189] Morgan RA et al. Case report of a serious adverse event following the administration of T cells transduced with a chimeric antigen receptor recognizing ERBB2. Molecular Therapy. 2010;**18**(4):843-851

[190] Brown CE et al. Bioactivity and safety of IL13Rα2-redirected chimeric antigen receptor CD8+ T cells in patients with recurrent glioblastoma. Clinical Cancer Research. 2015;**21**(18):4062-4072

[191] Katz SC et al. Phase I hepatic immunotherapy for metastases study of intra-arterial chimeric antigen receptor–modified T-cell therapy for CEA+ liver metastases. Clinical Cancer Research. 2015;**21**(14):3149-3159

[192] Wang L-CS et al. Targeting fibroblast activation protein in tumor stroma with chimeric antigen receptor T cells can inhibit tumor growth and augment host immunity without severe toxicity. Cancer Immunology Research. 2014;**2**(2):154-166

[193] Leko V, Rosenberg SA. Identifying and targeting human tumor antigens for T cell-based immunotherapy of solid tumors. Cancer Cell. 2020;**38**(4):454-472

[194] Shah NN, Fry TJ. Mechanisms of resistance to CAR T cell therapy. Nature Reviews Clinical Oncology. 2019;**16**(6):372-385

[195] Stroncek DF et al. Myeloid cells in peripheral blood mononuclear cell concentrates inhibit the expansion of chimeric antigen receptor T cells. Cytotherapy. 2016;**18**(7):893-901

[196] Okoye AA, Picker LJ. CD 4+ T-cell depletion in HIV infection: Mechanisms of immunological failure. Immunological Reviews. 2013;**254**(1):54-64

[197] Caulier B, Enserink JM, Wälchli S. Pharmacologic control of CAR T cells. International Journal of Molecular Sciences. 2021;**22**(9):4320

[198] Jacoby E. Relapse and resistance to CAR-T cells and Blinatumomab in hematologic malignancies. Clinical Hematology International. 2019;**1**(2):79-84

[199] Lopes AG, Noel R, Sinclair A. Cost analysis of vein-to-vein CAR T-cell therapy: Automated manufacturing and supply chain. Cell and Gene Therapy Insights. 2020;**6**(3):487-510

[200] Eyles JE et al. Cell therapy products: Focus on issues with manufacturing and quality control of chimeric antigen receptor T-cell therapies. Journal of Chemical Technology & Biotechnology. 2019;**94**(4):1008-1016

[201] Schuessler-Lenz M et al. Marketing regulatory oversight of advanced therapy medicinal products in Europe. In: Regulatory Aspects of Gene Therapy and Cell Therapy Products: A Global Perspective. Springer; 2023. pp. 1-21

[202] Krackhardt AM et al. Clinical translation and regulatory aspects of CAR/TCR-based adoptive cell therapies—The German cancer consortium approach. Cancer Immunology, Immunotherapy. 2018;**67**:513-523

[203] Hayakawa T et al. Report of the international regulatory forum on human cell therapy and gene therapy products. Biologicals. 2016;**44**(5):467-479

Chapter 6

Endocrine Adverse Events in Cancer Immunotherapy: From Mechanisms to Clinical Practice

Olexiy Aseyev, Alesha Bishop, Hannah Shortreed, Elycia Monaghan and Yue Sun

Abstract

Immunotherapy-induced endocrinopathies remain an adverse risk factor for patients undergoing PD-1/PD-L1 and CTLA-4 target immunotherapy treatment. Immunotherapy works by boosting the immune system to target, bind and block tumor receptors that would otherwise allow the cells to camouflage. This paper focuses on thyroid dysfunction, adrenal insufficiency, diabetes mellitus, and hypophysitis, and specifically the clinical presentation, diagnostic approaches, and management of each. All four endocrinopathies often present with generalized symptoms and, therefore, are commonly misdiagnosed. Healthcare professionals must closely monitor symptoms through laboratory testing and, when necessary, diagnostic imaging to appropriately diagnose and treat endocrinopathies. Thyroid dysfunction and adrenal insufficiency are often debated on immunotherapy hold/discontinuation. However, treatment of grade 3–4 diabetes mellitus and hypophysitis results in holding treatment until immune function prognosis decreases or returns to normal. Overall, ongoing research and clinical trials are needed to understand the varying effects of immunotherapy-induced endocrinopathies. Healthcare professionals should always consider patient symptoms, laboratory results and diagnostic imaging to ensure endocrinopathies are not missed and patients receive optimal care.

Keywords: cancer immunotherapy, endocrinopathies, diagnostic approaches, management strategies, adverse effects

1. Introduction

One cannot read about immunotherapy without encountering its unique history, with one individual coined as the "Father of Immunology", William B. Coley [1–3]. Coley is widely regarded as the first individual to endeavor to mobilize the immune system in treating cancer in the 1891, producing regression of tumor growth in patients with sarcoma by injecting inactivated *Streptococcus pyogenes* and *Serratia marcescens* [2]. These injections were later termed "Coley's toxins" [1, 3]. Another hallmark of immunotherapy is the initiation of IL-2 (AKA T cell growth factor) as the first cancer immunotherapy in humankind, with FDA approval in 1992 in treating renal cell carcinoma that has metastasized [1, 2].

Immunotherapy is a treatment that boosts the immune system's power to fight cancer [2]. It focuses on how cancer cells interact with our body's natural defense system [2–4]. It considers the complex relationship between tumor cells and immunosurveillance [4]. This interaction involves three key steps. First, our immune system, which has both innate and adaptive components, works to destroy cancer cells [1, 2]. Second, there's a dynamic balance between the actions of the immune system and cancer cells, where cancer cells adapt to resist the immune attack [2, 3]. Finally, cancer cells may evade detection by the immune system and continue to grow and spread [2, 4]. Immunotherapy is just in its early days, yet it has drastically altered the cancer treatment landscape [1, 3].

Immune checkpoints and their inhibition continue to be an integral part of immunotherapy [1–4]. Immune checkpoints are receptors found on the surface of T cells, and they serve as the gatekeeper of immune responses in terms of either propagation or inhibition [4–7]. This gatekeeping is in keeping with the process of immuno-editing, involving the immune system's ability to keep tumor growth at bay by modifying tumor immunogenicity or modulating tumor escape by decreasing anti-tumor defense responses, or even simultaneously [2]. The way in which immune checkpoints prevent autoimmune dysfunction is in the former option, where negative feedback plays a role in avoiding overactivation of T cells [5]. In the latter option, tumor cells exploit immune checkpoints to weaken the response from the immune system so that they can escape immune modulation and thereby proliferate [4]. Immune checkpoint inhibitors utilize antibodies to inhibit this gatekeeper to allow for antitumor activity [2].

2. Endocrinopathies

As with other treatments, immunotherapy can cause side effects [8]. Specifically, immune checkpoint inhibitors, a type of immunotherapy, are known to trigger immune-related adverse events (irAEs) [7, 8]. These include conditions like colitis, skin inflammation (dermatitis), liver inflammation (hepatitis), and various disorders related to hormone glands (endocrinopathies) [7, 8]. These inhibitors work by blocking certain immune checkpoint receptors, such as cytotoxic T-lymphocyte antigen 4 CTLA-4 and programmed cell death protein 1 (PD-1) or its ligand (PD-L1), to attack cancer cells [8]. However, this blocking can lead to an excessive immune response against normal cells, resulting in side effects ranging from mild to severe [8]. Detailed explanations of these processes are found in the following sections.

Research shows that about 10% of patients treated with immune checkpoint inhibitors experience endocrinopathies [8]. The most common are thyroid disorders and inflammation of the pituitary gland (hypophysitis) [8]. Less common are problems with the pancreas, adrenal, and parathyroid glands [7, 8]. It is important for both endocrinologists and oncologists to be aware of these potential side effects. Early identification of signs and symptoms, accurate diagnosis, and effective treatment strategies are crucial for successful patient outcomes [8].

2.1 Mechanisms of immunotherapy-induced endocrinopathies

Immunotherapy has become a revolutionary cancer treatment that utilizes the body's immune system to target and destroy malignant cells [7]. Immune checkpoints are specialized proteins on the surface of immune cells that communicate with T cells to prevent cell destruction [6]. Some tumor cells present this unique mechanism to impersonate normal immune cells [3]. As T cells checkpoint different cells, tumor cells with the required proteins bind to the T cell receptors and bypass destruction [3, 4]. However, immunotherapy inhibits the ability of tumor cells to camouflage by blocking the checkpoint connection [4, 5]. Therefore, the T cell recognizes the tumor cell as a pathogen and initiates cell death [6]. A significant downside of checkpoint inhibitor immunotherapy is its impact on endocrine function [7, 8]. The focus in current research is on two checkpoint inhibitors: PD-1 and its associated protein PD-L1, and CTLA-4 [4, 5, 7]. However, when these checkpoints are blocked by immunotherapy, it leads to increased immune activity [1]. Such an increase can result in autoimmune dysfunction, whereby the immune system mistakenly attacks healthy cells and organs [9].

2.1.1 PD-1/PD-L1

Programmed Cell Death Protein 1 (PD-1) is a receptor commonly associated with immune cells, including T cells used in late immune response [6, 9]. PD-1 co-protein Programmed Cell Death Ligand 1 (PD-L1) receptor is found on tumor cells [6, 9]. The prevalence of PD-L1 receptors is more commonly associated with solid cancers [5]. The mechanism of action results in the binding of PD-1 to PD-L1, therefore labelling the tumor cell as non-pathogenic and therefore, no T cell activation or proliferation of cytotoxic activity occurs [5]. In addition, the PD-1/PD-L1 binding may initiate apoptosis of the T cell, establishing a greater immune tolerance [10]. Overall, the PD-1/PD-L1 receptor binding enables the tumor cell to mimic a healthy cell, escaping an immune response and continuing to proliferate [5, 10]. Immune checkpoint inhibitors overcome these mechanisms by individually binding to PD-1 and PD-L1 receptors, preventing the direct binding of PD-1/PD-L1 depicted in **Figure 1** [5, 9] . Without the direct binding of PD-1/PD-L1, the T cell receptor binds to the antigen receptor located on the tumor cell, which is now recognized as a pathogen [5]. The T cell proliferates, surrounds the tumor cell, and releases granzymes or pore-forming proteins to trigger cell death [1, 5].

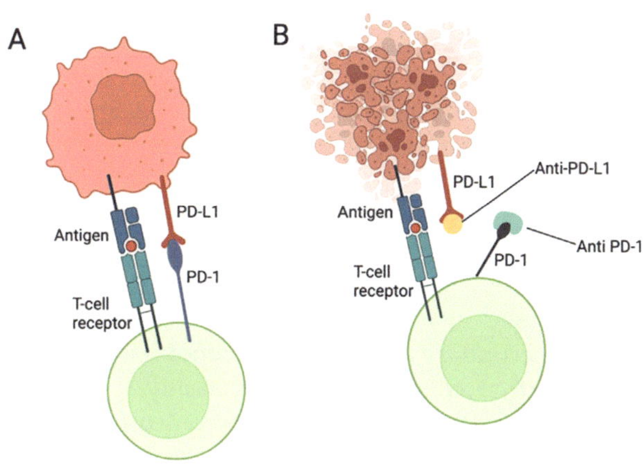

Figure 1.
(A) PD-1/PD-L1 binding to inhibit T cell activation. (B) PD-1/PD-L1 checkpoint inhibitors preventing binding and therefore T cell activation occurs [11].

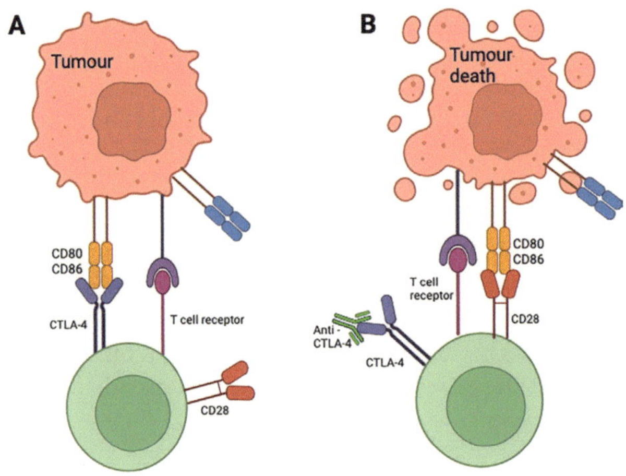

Figure 2.
(A) CTLA-4 binding to CD80/CD86 inhibiting T cell. (B) Anti CTLA-4 checkpoint inhibitor, binding to CTLA-4, allowing for CD28 to bind to CD80/CD86 resulting in T cell proliferation and tumor death [13].

2.1.2 CTLA-4

Cytotoxic T-lymphocyte-associated antigen 4 (CTLA-4) is an endocytic molecule found on the surface of specific T cells that regulate early T cell proliferation [12]. The binding of CTLA-4 to distinct ligands, CD80 and CD86, located on the tumor cell, can inhibit the activation of T cells [12]. Immunotherapy CTLA-4 checkpoint inhibitors block the binding of CTLA-4 and CD80/CD86, allowing the T cell to proliferate and destroy the tumor cell, pictured in **Figure 2** [12].

3. Types of endocrinopathies

3.1 Thyroid dysfunction

10% of all patients experience endocrinopathies secondary to checkpoint inhibitors [9]. Thyroid dysfunction is the most prevalent endocrinopathy for patients undergoing PD-1 and CTLA-4 inhibitors, with more significant onset associated with PD-1 [9]. The epidemiology of thyroid dysfunction secondary to immunotherapy is limited [11]. However, thyroiditis presents as a common pathology, potentially arising from PD-1/CTLA-4 disrupting normal thyroid function, resulting in an immune response triggering hypothyroidism or hyperthyroidism [14].

3.1.1 Clinical presentation

Thyroid dysfunction secondary to immune checkpoint inhibitors may present as Hypothyroidism or Hyperthyroidism [11, 14]. Commonly, signs and symptoms of immunotherapy-induced hypothyroidism/hyperthyroidism demonstrate similarities to primary thyroid dysfunction [11]. Hypothyroidism occurs from an underactive thyroid gland, resulting in symptoms including bradycardia, weight gain, constipation, and fatigue [9, 14]. Hyperthyroidism, or thyrotoxicosis, manifests as tachycardia, weight loss, diarrhea, and fatigue and is a consequence of an overactive thyroid gland [9, 14]. It is important to note that these symptoms are representative and often dismissed as other illnesses relating to immunotherapy [9]. Careful analysis should take place when a patient is experiencing subtle or severe symptoms [9]. Hypothyroidism presents more often, with the onset of 71 days with PD-1 alone and 63 days with combined therapy [11, 14]. Hyperthyroidism is less common but still noted, with an onset of 47 days after initial treatment on PD-1 monotherapy and 21 days for combination therapy [11, 14].

3.1.1.1 Case Vignette

An 81-year-old female diagnosed with metastatic lung cancer treated with carboplatin and pemetrexed and four cycles of pembrolizumab immunotherapy presented to the emergency department with symptoms of weakness and fatigue resulting in a near-fall. The patient denied symptoms of nausea, headaches, diarrhea or weight gain. Other than hypertension, the patient's past medical history is unremarkable. Laboratory results presented an elevated TSH of 178 (normal range = 0.4–4.0 mlU/L) and a free T4 of less than 1 (normal range = 0.9–1.9 ng/dl). Sodium, potassium, chloride, and bicarbonate were all within normal range. Urinalysis was positive for leukocytes and white blood cells. Based on elevated TSH levels, the patient was diagnosed with pembrolizumab-induced hypothyroidism. The thyroid dysfunction presented 3–4 months after initiating pembrolizumab, corresponding with the literature's onset of 63–71 days. The patient was treated with 50 mcg of oral levothyroxine and prednisone due to significant symptoms and elevated laboratory values. TSH was repeated in 6 weeks. The patient did not receive any diagnostic imaging, most likely due to the severely elevated TSH level used as an indication to begin treatment. Antibodies were also ordered to rule out Hashimoto's Thyroiditis. The patients' TSH values decreased after 6 weeks, and they could continue pembrolizumab treatment.

- Adapted from our clinical case.

3.1.2 Diagnostic approaches

The detection of thyroid issues, such as hyperthyroidism or hypothyroidism, might not always start with obvious symptoms [6, 14]. It is recommended that patients undergo baseline blood tests before starting immunotherapy [14]. These tests provide a reference point, helping doctors identify any changes in thyroid function that might occur during treatment [6]. Baseline blood tests that should be performed include complete blood count (CBC), comprehensive metabolic panel (CMP), thyroid-stimulating Hormone (TSH) (normal range between 0.4 and 4.0 mlU/L), free thyroxine (T4) (total T4 = 0.4–2.5 mlU/l, FreeT4 = 0.9–1.9 ng/dl), Triiodothyronine (total T3) (0.9–2.8 nmol/L) and urinalysis for baseline kidney function (GFR ≥60) [15]; Liver function test (LFT) may also be considered as part of baseline measurements [15]. Adrenal insufficiency should be ruled out, as symptoms present similar to thyroid dysfunction [15]. Underlying medical conditions, including Hashimoto's or Graves's Disease, may produce thyroid antibodies that affect the overall function of the thyroid gland [1]. If a patient's medical or family history demonstrates a risk for autoimmune disorders, physicians should consider performing a thyroid peroxidase antibody test (TPO) to rule out potential comorbidities that may present as thyroid dysfunction [15].

Hyperthyroidism secondary to immunotherapy diagnostically presents with a TSH below 0.4 mlU/L, whereas hypothyroidism presents with a TSH greater than 4.0 mlU/L [15]. A baseline Electrocardiogram (ECG) would provide important information if the patient has previous or is at risk of cardiovascular complications [15]. If thyroid dysfunction is symptomatic with positive lab results, a thyroid ultrasound or radioactive thyroid uptake scan can be performed (except in the case of pregnancy) to determine if the thyroid gland is underactive or hyperactive [15].

Laboratory results should be interpreted considering potential factors, including steroid use, iodine contrast, and non-thyroid illnesses [16].

3.1.3 Management strategies

Medical interventions for patients experiencing thyroid dysfunction secondary to immunotherapy should be constructed with an individualistic approach [11]. For patients experiencing hyperthyroidism, beta-blockers and antithyroid medications are commonly prescribed [11]. When treating hypothyroidism with an elevated TSH (specifically TSH $>$ 10 mU/L) and symptom presentation, initiating hormone replacement medication is shown to have a high overall survival rate [1, 2]. Levothyroxine (1–1.6 mcg/kg/day) is a first-line treatment and works by replacing the thyroxine hormone that is under-produced by the thyroid gland [14]. Before administering levothyroxine, age and comorbidities should be considered. Other medications used for managing hypothyroidism include propranolol and atenolol [11].

After establishing baseline blood work and diagnostic imaging, TSH and FreeT4 are recommended every 4–8 weeks while receiving immunotherapy and every 3–6 months post-treatment [2, 14, 16]. In patients with diagnosed hyperthyroidism, TSH should be monitored every 2–3 weeks until laboratory results increase or until persistent hyperthyroidism can be established and treated [14]. It is important to note that patients with hyperthyroidism are at increased risk for developing hypothyroidism due to ongoing thyroiditis [15]. For patients experiencing hypothyroidism, TSH should be completed every 6–8 weeks [14]. In addition, cytokines and other inflammatory markers have been associated with tissue damage and inflammatory response, impacting thyroid function [14]. Monitoring inflammatory markers is essential in the early detection of thyroid dysfunction and maintaining regular thyroid activity [11].

In the case of thyroid dysfunction, discontinuing immunotherapy is deemed unnecessary unless the patient is severely symptomatic [1, 14]. In this case, immunotherapy should be held until symptoms resolve [14]. There are no known immunotherapy dose reduction recommendations regarding thyroid dysfunction [15]. Hyperthyroidism and hypothyroidism with respective symptoms and diagnostic implications are shown in **Figure 3**.

3.2 Adrenal insufficiency

Adrenal insufficiency (AI) is an endocrine adverse event that can occur with the use of immune checkpoint inhibitors (**Figure 4**) [17–20]. AI is a particularly salient adverse event as it is often misdiagnosed and therefore not always treated [17, 19]. It is important to differentiate between primary adrenal insufficiency (PAI) and secondary adrenal insufficiency (SAI), with the former being relatively rare and due to lack of glucocorticoid and/or mineralocorticoid production from the adrenal gland cortex [17–19]. PAI can possibly be lethal, as glucocorticoids and mineralocorticoids have essential roles in homeostasis of sodium, fluids, and energy [18]. SAI is related to inflammation within

DOI: http://dx.doi.org/10.5772/intechopen.1004625

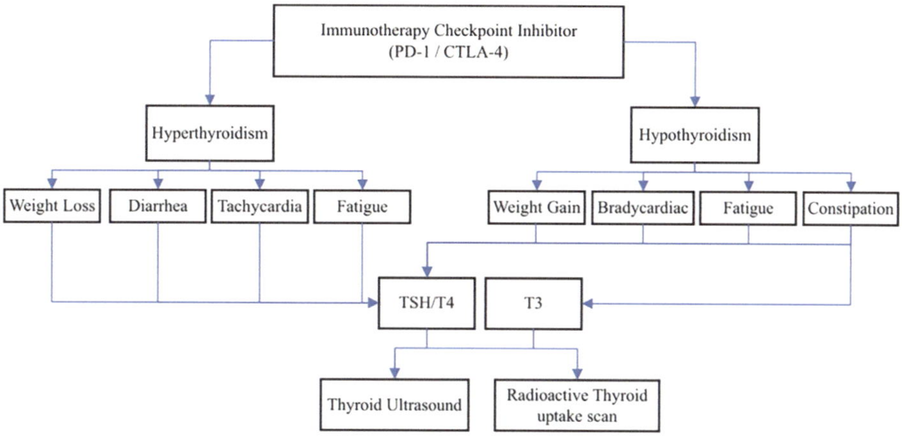

Figure 3.
Representation of thyroid dysfunction, with presenting symptoms, laboratory testing and diagnostic imaging.

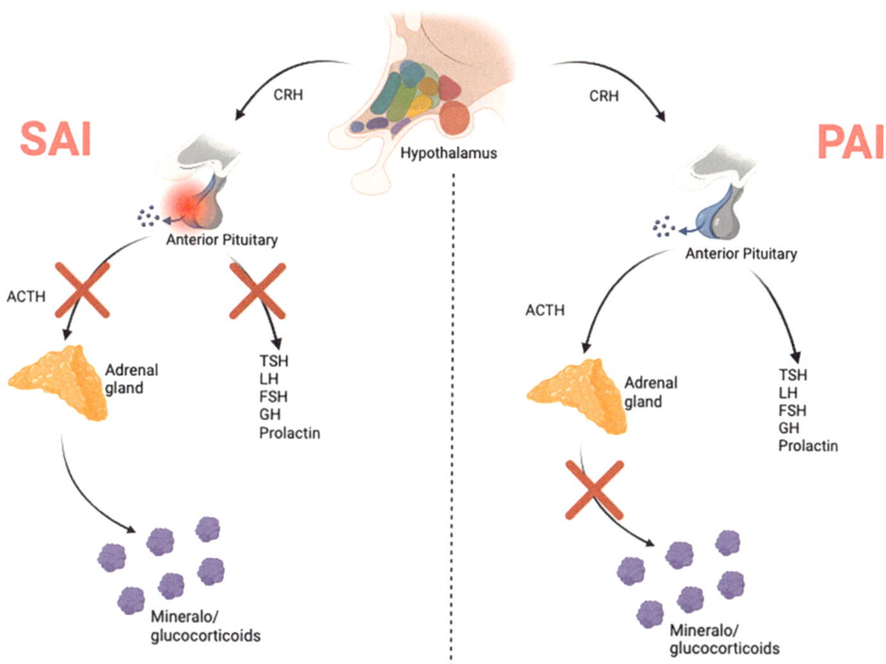

Figure 4.
Pathophysiology of PAI versus SAI. PAI is due to the lack of mineralocorticoids and glucocorticoids being released from the adrenal gland. SAI is due to inflammation within the anterior pituitary, thereby causing decreased ACTH release along with possible decrease of other anterior pituitary hormones, including TSH, LH, FSH, GH, and prolactin [17].

the pituitary gland, leading to diminished adrenocorticotropic hormone (ACTH) production and therefore loss of cortisol release [17–19]. Although not immediately life threatening, it may possibly impact other hormones produced by the anterior pituitary, including luteinizing hormone (LH), follicle-stimulating hormone (FSH), growth hormone, prolactin, and thyroid-stimulating hormone (TSH) [17].

3.2.1 Clinical presentation

Patients with both PAI and SAI present with non-specific symptoms such as orthostatic hypotension, nausea and vomiting, weakness, fatigue, and abdominal pain [17–20]. One sign more so specific to SAI is eosinophilia due to the active inflammatory response within the anterior pituitary [18]. Other laboratory abnormalities include hyponatremia, hypoglycemia [18–20], hyperkalemia, and decreased morning levels of cortisol [17, 19, 20]. If a patient is experiencing an acute adrenal crisis, they may present with fever, confusion, lethargy, and anorexia [17, 19]. Cases of AI induced by immune checkpoint inhibitors have been observed in 1–2% of patients after receiving either anti-PD-1 or anti-PD-1 combined with CTLA-4 therapy, with this varying depending on types of cancer and immunotherapy being received [19]. AI can also present as syncope along with other non-specific symptoms, which is illustrated by the below case study [17].

3.2.1.1 Case Vignette

Mr. O is a 67-year-old male with metastatic melanoma with various skin lesions and nodules within his axillary lymph nodes and torso. This patient's past medical history is significant for hypertension, hyperlipidemia, and cerebral vascular accident. Mr. O had received four doses of ipilimumab and nivolumab for treatment of metastatic melanoma. Following his most recent dose of these two immunotherapy agents, PET/CT scan had shown an increase in the amount and size of cutaneous lesions. About 7 days later, this patient started to report gastrointestinal symptoms including nausea and constipation, for which he was prescribed a proton pump inhibitor (PPI). This intervention allowed for improvement of his nausea, but soon after Mr. O had presented to the emergency department following a syncopal episode. After blood work had been ordered, he was noted to have hyponatremia and hypokalemia, for which he received intravenous fluids. This however did little to improve his sodium levels, and Mr. O was later found to have syndrome of inappropriate antidiuretic hormone (SIADH). After this diagnosis had been made, he was given sodium tablets and later discharged home with stable serum sodium levels.

- Adapted from Martella et al. [19].

3.2.2 Diagnostic approaches

Laboratory tests to assist in the diagnosis of AI include cortisol and ACTH drawn in the morning, along with ACTH stimulation testing to assess for the extent of adrenal insufficiency [17, 18, 20]. In terms of morning cortisol, results consistent with adrenal insufficiency are low morning cortisol, as normal physiology has it so that cortisol levels are normally increased in the morning in accordance with normal circadian rhythms [19]. To distinguish between primary and secondary adrenal insufficiency, morning ACTH levels are usually increased in PAI as a result of the anterior pituitary's reaction to decreased cortisol prediction from the adrenal gland [20]. Another PAI result would be a diminished aldosterone serum concentration, along with hyponatremia and hyperkalemia [17, 18]; this differs from SAI, where one would expect to see low or normal TSH levels and decreased free thyroxine levels [17, 18].

One imaging modality that would be particularly helpful in ruling out other conditions would be a CT of the head, which would assist in assessing for metastatic spread or hemorrhage [17]. Other imaging that can be ordered includes an MRI of the head/hypophysis, where in SAI the pituitary stalk would be noted as increased in size or the pituitary gland itself would be enhanced [17, 18, 20]. This can be performed with or without contrast and would be indicated in patients with new symptoms of increased intracranial pressure, including new onset severe headaches and visual changes [17]. In terms of imaging the adrenal glands, CT of these structures may assist in the diagnosis of PAI, possibly showing smoothened contours of the glands which would indicate elevated volumes [20].

3.2.3 Management strategies

The main treatment for AI, regardless of it being primary or secondary, is corticosteroids [17, 18, 20]. If symptoms are acute, hydrocortisone is the medication of choice, with the first dose being 100 mg administered intravenously as a form of physiologic stress dosing [17, 20]. Following this, the dose would be tapered down to 50 mg given every 6–8 hours, followed by another taper of 10–20 mg given in the morning and another 5–10 mg given in the early afternoon [17]. Cautious consideration should be given in administering high dose corticosteroids such as methylprednisolone or prednisone 1 mg/kg/day as there are several studies noting an association between high dose corticosteroids and increased mortality [17].

There is debate as to whether one should discontinue taking immune checkpoint inhibitors if AI occurs [17, 20]. One source notes that they should be stopped in all patients with AI [20], while another reference suggests holding immune checkpoint inhibitors until the patient is clinically stable or in patients that have a diagnosis that is ambiguous [17]. Corticosteroids may have to be discontinued as well as they may lead to decreased ACTH, causing amplified AI symptoms [18]. The corticosteroid of choice is usually hydrocortisone [17, 20]. Accompanying this, treatment of additional symptoms slightly differs in cases of PAI versus SAI, with PAI requiring treatment of mineralocorticoid deficiency using fludrocortisone, which will also assist with recovery of hyponatremia and hypotension [17, 20]. SAI, due to its effects on the anterior pituitary, may also result in central hypothyroidism, necessitating use of thyroid replacement therapy [17, 18]. This must be done with consideration of mitigating the risk of adrenal crisis, which involves starting corticosteroids before starting thyroid hormone replacement [17]. Monitoring therapy of SAI should involve evaluating free T4 as opposed to TSH [17]. It should be noted that AI may be a lifelong condition for most patients, however with recovery from AI symptoms and continuation of maintenance therapy, patients may safely continue with ICI therapy [17].

3.3 Diabetes mellitus

Of the documented endocrinopathies secondary to initiation of immunotherapy, pancreatic endocrine dysfunction is less common but can lead to life-threatening complications such as rapid-onset diabetic ketoacidosis (DKA) [8]. The use of immune checkpoint inhibitors, such as PD-1 and its associated ligand PD-L1, is associated with a 0.2–0.9% incidence of diabetes mellitus (DM) [21]. This includes both new-onset type 1 DM (T1DM) and worsening type-2 DM (T2DM) [8]. The pathophysiology of immunotherapy-induced pancreatic endocrine dysfunction appears to mirror the autoimmune destruction seen with T1DM but with more rapid T-cell-mediated destruction of pancreatic β-cells [8]. The exact mechanisms involved in this process are poorly understood; one pathway, describing PD-1/PD-L1 regulation of

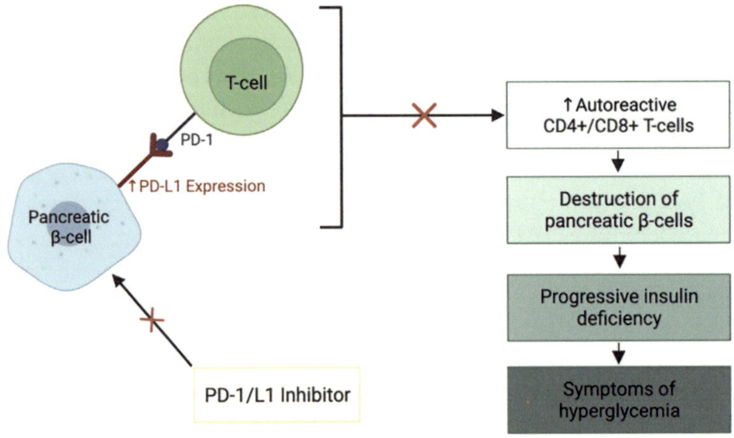

Figure 5.
Proposed pathogenesis of diabetes mellitus (DM) secondary to initiation of therapy with immune checkpoint inhibitors. Under normal conditions, pancreatic β-cells express PD-L1, preventing them from being subjected to immune destruction [22]. It has been hypothesized that β-cells can attenuate the immune response in pancreatic islets through upregulation of PD-L1 expression, as seen in patients with T1DM [22]. Immune checkpoint inhibitors that target PD-1 and PD-L1 may, therefore, disrupt this process, leading to activation of autoreactive CD4+ and CD8+ T-cells, destruction of β-cells in the pancreatic islets, progressive insulin deficiency, and subsequent hyperglycemia characteristic of DM [22].

T-cell activation, provides some insight into this process and is depicted in **Figure 5** [22]. This pathway has been observed and replicated in mouse models and observed indirectly in human studies involving patients with T1DM [22]. Alternative pathways involve the development of autoimmune DM antibodies and CTLA-4 regulation of T-cell activation [22]. However, half of all patients who develop DM secondary to initiation of immunotherapy are found to be autoantibody negative and expression of CTLA-4 in islet cells is unconfirmed, making these pathways more uncertain [22]. Moreover, 70% of patients who develop T1DM secondary to initiation of immunotherapy have a genetic predisposition to DM, suggesting that genetic linkage may play a role in the underlying pathophysiology [8].

3.3.1 Clinical presentation

New-onset or worsening DM secondary to immunotherapy has been observed in many patients [7]. Clinically, patients can present with symptoms of thirst, polydipsia, polyuria, weight loss, dehydration, and lethargy [8]. Roughly two-thirds of patients can present with DKA, while the remainder suffers from severe hyperglycemia (both insulin-dependent and non-insulin-dependent) [7, 8]. The median time to onset of signs and symptoms following the initiation of immunotherapy typically occurs between 7 and 17 weeks [8]. A few cases have demonstrated that it can take years for evidence of pancreatic endocrine dysfunction to become apparent, while in others, signs and symptoms might appear sooner than 7 weeks, as shown in the Case Vignette [8, 23].

3.3.1.1 Case Vignette

A 73-year-old man with no personal history or family history of diabetes mellitus developed stage IV M1c metastatic melanoma. He was initially treated with vemurafenib, a BRAF inhibitor, and cobimetinib, a MEK inhibitor. After 3 months, his disease had progressed, and a second-line therapy with nivolumab, a PD-1 inhibitor, was initiated at 3 mg/kg every 2 weeks. After 6 weeks of treatment with nivolumab, the patient presented to the emergency department with sudden onset vomiting, abdominal pain, and severe asthenia, which were found to be associated with polyuria-polydipsia syndrome. Investigations revealed the following: glycemia: 27.78 mmol/l; bicarbonate: 18 mmol/l; urinary dipstick test positive for glucose and ketone; creatinine: 177 μmol/l; and glycated hemoglobin (HbA_{1c}): 8.8%. These findings, considering his clinical presentation, were consistent with diabetic ketoacidosis (DKA) resulting from the onset of type 1 diabetes mellitus with acute renal failure. Insulin therapy was initiated, and nivolumab was withheld for 3.5 weeks. This was successful in normalizing his glycemia and alleviating his clinical symptoms. Subsequent laboratory investigations revealed the presence of islet cell autoantibodies (anti-glutamic acid decarboxylase antibody, zinc transporter 8 antibody, and protein phosphatase-like and insulinoma antigen-2 antibody), while C-peptide was undetectable. Retrospective investigations of frozen serum stored at 0 weeks and 3 months before initiating nivolumab treatment showed the presence of these islet cell autoantibodies, while insulin, C-peptide concentrations, and glycemia were found to be normal. The same dose of nivolumab was resumed after 3.5 weeks with no further effects on glycemia. After 3 months of treatment with nivolumab, the tumor showed a complete metabolic response on imaging. In the context of the investigations before and after initiation of treatment with nivolumab and the patient's clinical presentation, this case report highlights the autoimmune origin of diabetes secondary to treatment with a PD-1 inhibitor in a predisposed patient.

- Adapted from Gauci et al. [24].

3.3.2 Diagnostic approaches

In patients receiving therapy with immune checkpoint inhibitors and presenting with symptoms of new-onset or worsening DM (i.e. polydipsia, polyuria, nausea, and vomiting, etc.,) investigations should include testing for elevated plasma glucose, low or absent C-peptide, and mildly elevated glycated hemoglobin (HbA_{1c}) [8, 25]. The diagnostic criteria for DM in Canada stipulate that a single laboratory test result in the diabetes range (i.e. random plasma glucose $\geq$11.1 mmol/L or HbA1c $\geq$ 6.5%) is diagnostic in the presence of symptomatic hyperglycemia [26]. Conversely, in the absence of symptomatic hyperglycemia, a single laboratory test result in the diabetes range requires repeat confirmatory testing (fasting plasma glucose, oral glucose tolerance test, and HbA_{1c}) on a separate day to diagnose DM [26].

Detection of autoantibodies, such as anti-glutamic acid decarboxylase (GAD) and anti-islet cell (ICA), can be used to distinguish between T1DM and T2DM [8, 26]. Of note, autoantibodies are positive in nearly half of patients and may precede or coincide with their development of T1DM [8, 26]. Additionally, in the absence of autoantibodies, T1DM should not be ruled out, as autoantibody levels can vary over time and lack the diagnostic accuracy to necessitate routine use [26]. Alternative autoantibodies for the diagnosis of T1DM include zinc transporter 8, protein phosphatase-like, and insulinoma antigen-2 [24].

Imaging in diagnosing DM secondary to immunotherapy is restricted to non-specific signs, including pancreatic enlargement, pancreatic atrophy, and findings that mirror diffuse pancreatitis [22]. Furthermore, imaging for the diagnosis of DM is not recognized in Canadian diagnostic guidelines, further indicating its limited use as a diagnostic modality [26].

3.3.3 Management strategies

All patients planning to undergo immunotherapy with immune checkpoint inhibitors should be informed of their DM risk and receive education on the warning signs for hyperglycemia and DKA before initiating treatment [22]. Care providers must also be aware of this risk and pursue the necessary diagnostic tests (i.e., plasma glucose, HbA_{1c}, ketones, blood gases, etc.) if DM or DKA is suspected based on the patient's clinical presentation [22]. Monitoring plasma glucose and HbA_{1c} before initiating treatment and during treatment as a follow-up should also be performed to ensure that the presentation of DM is caught early, and treatment regimens are modified accordingly [22].

In the context of DM secondary to the initiation of immunotherapy, presentation of DKA should be managed according to standard methods (i.e. fluid resuscitation, potassium repletion, etc.) and discontinuation of immunotherapy is recommended until DKA is resolved [7, 22]. Patients whose DKA has been resolved or who have new onset hyperglycemia in the absence of DKA can adhere to treatment recommendations based on their grade of hyperglycemia (as defined by the Common Terminology Criteria for Adverse Events (CTCAE) grading system) [22]. In short, for patients with grade 1 hyperglycemia, immunotherapy may be continued with close laboratory monitoring and without the initiation of insulin therapy [22]. For patients with grade 2 hyperglycemia, immunotherapy can be continued, though insulin therapy should be started to manage clinical symptoms [8, 22]. In patients whose hyperglycemia is a grade 3 or 4, immunotherapy should be withheld, and insulin therapy should be initiated to mitigate the effects of progressive pancreatic endocrine dysfunction [22]. Immunotherapy should be withheld until symptoms and laboratory values are returned to grade 1; at this point, re-administration of immunotherapeutic agents can be considered with close monitoring of blood glucose levels [22]. Moreover, for patients with worsening T2DM after starting immunotherapy, evidence suggests that immunotherapy can continue uninterrupted with additional consideration given to oral antihyperglycemic agents, lifestyle counseling, and vascular complication management [8].

Notably, treatment with glucocorticoid has the potential to worsen pancreatic endocrine dysfunction and exacerbate symptoms of hyperglycemia [7, 8]. This contrasts with the treatment of other immune-related adverse events, including hepatotoxicity and colitis, as glucocorticoids can have adverse effects on blood glucose levels and should, therefore, be avoided in the setting of DM secondary to the initiation of immunotherapy [7, 8, 22].

Finally, management should include referral to a diabetes team and a system to ensure safe and continuous access to insulin for those requiring insulin treatment [7]. Initial patient education through a diabetes specialist is also recommended [7]. DM secondary to the initiation of immunotherapy is generally irreversible, so such measures are necessary to ensure the well-being of patients with this diagnosis [22].

3.4 Hypophysitis

Hypophysitis is induced when the pituitary gland is inflamed due to varied hormone dysfunction [27]. It is a well-established irAE [27]. Variable incidence has been reported in patients treated with immune checkpoint inhibitors [27, 28]. Higher irAE incidence is associated with the male gender, older age, and higher treatment dose [27]. High incidence is also associated with high-dose anti-CTLA-4 inhibitors, ipilimumab, treatment (>3 mg) at 17%, whereas a lower incidence of up to 1% has been reported for patients treated with anti-PD-1/PD-L1 inhibitors [27].

Hypophysitis induced by anti-CTLA-4 is mediated through type II and type IV hypersensitivity and the immune system [27]. More studies are needed about the pathogenesis of anti-PD-1/PD-L1 induced hypophysitis. In contrast to anti-CTLA-4, which affects various pituitary cells equally, anti-PD-1/PD-L1-induced hypophysitis targets ACTH-secreting cells [27]. One proposed mechanism is autoimmunity against corticotrophs and ectopic expression of ACTH in tumors [27]. Preliminary studies suggest hypothalamic autoimmunity as a reason for developing pituitary dysfunction in patients treated with anti-PD-1/PD-L1 [27].

3.4.1 Clinical presentation

There is a wide range of onset times after the initiation of immune checkpoint inhibitors [27, 28]. In general, anti-CLTA-induced hypophysitis presents earlier in treatment than hypophysitis due to anti-PD-1/PD-L1 [27]. For example, in patients treated with ipilimumab, the median time to onset is 9–11 weeks with a range of 1–35 weeks, and the median time to onset for pembrolizumab is 16 weeks with a range of 1–52 weeks [27]. The presenting symptoms for immune checkpoint inhibitor-induced adverse reactions are usually not specific, which include nausea, vomiting, reduced appetite, headache, and dizziness [27, 28]. A large proportion of patients can be asymptomatic at the time of diagnosis [27, 28]. There is an overlap of symptoms with hypopituitarism and that of the underlying malignancy, which adds challenges to diagnosis [28]. Patients on anti-PD-1/PD-L1 usually present with isolated ACTH deficiency without pituitary enlargement [27]. Patients with anti-CTLA-4-induced hypophysitis have more diverse presentations, including symptoms of hypothyroidism, hypogonadism, and visual disturbances [27].

3.4.1.1 Case Vignette

A 33-year-old female diagnosed with metastatic melanoma with involvement of pelvic and inguinal adenopathy and metastasis to the adrenal glands was treated with Ipilimumab/Nivolumab combination therapy. The diagnosis was established with an inguinal lymph node biopsy and PET scan; a repeat PET scan showed the patient's partial response to treatment. Sixty-four days after treatment initiation, the patient experienced headache, fatigue, palpitations, and joint pains. Laboratory evaluation showed TSH < 0.015mIU/mL (reference range 0.35–3.6), T4 16 mcg/dL (reference range 4.0–11.0), T3 235 ng/dL (58–160) concerning primary hyperthyroidism. Morning cortisol level was 10.8 mcg/dL (3.7–19.4) at the time, which was inconclusive for the diagnosis of adrenal insufficiency. MRI was performed due to worsening headache, which found pituitary gland enlargement with extension into the suprasellar space consistent with hypophysitis. This resulted in cessation of treatment, and the patient was treated with atenolol and prednisone 1 mg/kg/day tapered to 10 mg/day over 10 days. The patient's symptoms had significantly improved. A repeat MRI showed that the finding associated with hypophysitis had resolved. The patient's thyroid function returned to normal within 8 weeks. However, she was found to have adrenal insufficiency with undetectable morning cortisol during steroid taper and needed hydrocortisone replacement (15 g daily in divided doses). She was kept on nivolumab maintenance therapy after. Six years later, there was a recurrence of the melanoma, and the patient was rechallenged with Ipilimumab/nivolumab; she started to have symptoms, including headaches, nausea, and tachycardia 33 days after treatment initiation, and MRI again showed findings concerning hypophysitis. The patient was again successfully treated for hypophysitis with high-dose prednisone followed by hydrocortisone maintenance. Symptoms recurred after starting nivolumab maintenance therapy, and immunotherapy was stopped.

- Adapted from Park et al. [28].

3.4.2 Diagnostic approaches

Diagnosis or immune checkpoint inhibitor-induced endocrinopathies can be challenging due to variability in symptom onset and overlapping signs and symptoms with adverse reactions from concomitant treatment and malignancy itself [27]. Patients should be monitored for signs of hypophysitis, including headache, visual disturbances, fatigue, gastrointestinal symptoms, and hypotension [27]. Biochemical surveillance of hormone levels is important for diagnosing endocrine adverse reactions [27]. Laboratory investigations for monitoring of pituitary toxicity include TSH, free T4, morning ACTH and cortisol, prolactin, HbA1C, IGF-1, FSH, LH, and testosterone for males and estradiol for premenopausal females [11, 27]. Repeat laboratory investigations can be conducted regularly every 4–6 weeks during immunotherapy and every 6–12 after immunotherapy completion [11, 27]. Electrolytes and fasting glucose are also helpful for diagnostic evaluation [27]. On the rare occasion of suspected diabetes insipidus, serum and urine osmolality should be obtained [23, 27]. A pituitary MRI is recommended for evaluation if there is an abnormality with laboratory investigations to assess for hypophysitis versus metastatic disease [23, 27, 28].

3.4.3 Management strategies

Treatment for hypophysitis depends on the hormone affected and toxicity grade [23]. Treatment mainly involves holding immunotherapy, starting steroids and hormone replacement therapy, close follow up and monitoring [23]. Central adrenal insufficiency is the most common [23]. Patients could also develop central hypothyroidism, diabetes insipidus, hypogonadism and growth hormone deficiency [23]. For Grade 1 (asymptomatic or mild symptoms) and Grade 2 (moderate symptoms, able to perform ADL) toxicity, clinicians may consider holding treatment until the patient is stabilized on hormone replacement therapy [25]. Treatment should be held for Grades 3 and 4 (severe symptoms, medically significant) hypophysitis until stabilization [13, 25].

For patients with primary adrenal insufficiency and hypophysitis, 15–25 mg hydrocortisone in 2–3 divided doses is recommended for hormone replacement therapy [25]. High-dose glucocorticoid (hydrocortisone 100 mg intravenously followed by 50 mg every 6 hours) should be reserved for the treatment of adrenal crisis or compression symptoms from hypophysitis and the pituitary gland [23]. Thyroid hormones should be replaced in symptomatic patients with TSH elevation or asymptomatic patients with TSH levels that persist above 10mIU/L measured 4 weeks apart [23]. TSH should be monitored every 6 weeks while titrating too normal [23]. If thyroid hormone and corticosteroids are both required, the latter should be started several days earlier to prevent precipitation of adrenal crisis [23]. Replacement of gonadal hormones is recommended in men and women of reproductive age and is not advised in the setting of a poor oncologic prognosis [23]. In hypophysitis with active malignancy, growth hormone deficiency should not be treated [23]. Desmopressin is recommended for patients with hypophysitis and confirmed diabetic insipidus [23]. Endocrinopathy may be irreversible and may result in a need for lifelong hormone replacement [23, 28]. Endocrinology consultation is recommended in all cases [23, 28].

3.5 Other (hypogonadism, hypercalcemia)

In addition to central hypogonadism, as seen in hypophysitis, rare cases of immune checkpoint inhibitor-induced primary hypogonadism have been described [29]. WHO database for safety report, VigiBase recorded 13 cases of hypogonadism, and one case was primary hypogonadism [29]. A case study reported the development of bilateral orchitis with ipilimumab/nivolumab treatment, with laboratory investigations showing primary hypogonadism; this adverse reaction resolved without treatment and did not recur with future cycles [13]. This demonstrates that there is the potential for ICI to impact fertility and should be taken into consideration when treating patients of reproductive age.

Hypercalcemia is another adverse reaction of ICI therapy, which occurs via a variety of mechanisms [30]. It could occur due to immune checkpoint inhibitor-induced hyperparathyroidism or in the setting of thyroid dysfunction or adrenal insufficiency [30]. There are reports of hypercalcemia as a result of immune checkpoint inhibitor-induced sarcoid-like granulomas [30]. Furthermore, other reports show hypercalcemia associated with increased production of PTHrP and calcitriol [30]. This is a significant adverse reaction to recognize, as it could be confused with malignancy progression.

4. Prognostic implications

The prognosis of various endocrinopathies secondary to initiation of immunotherapy varies depending on which endocrine organ is involved [8]. This is documented with immune checkpoint inhibitors, wherein the thyroid, pituitary, pancreas, and adrenal glands can all be adversely impacted [8]. With thyroid dysfunction, the typical progression of disease occurs within 3–6 weeks, beginning initially with symptoms of hyperthyroidism and culminating in prolonged hypothyroidism [31]. Moreover, hyperthyroidism rarely persists and does not require additional therapy [8, 31]. However, for patients who develop hypothyroidism, long-term thyroid hormone replacement might be necessary for up to two-thirds of patients [8, 31]. Interestingly, hypothyroidism could benefit tumor progression in humans, such as improved response to treatment and increased progression-free survival [31]. However, further evidence is required to help define the role of findings in routine clinical practice [31].

Regarding pituitary dysfunction and hypophysitis, secondary adrenal insufficiency is considered irreversible, and the balance between high-dose glucocorticoid therapy and continued immunotherapy needs to be carefully monitored to ensure best patient outcomes [31]. As with hypothyroidism, several pieces of evidence suggest that patients who develop hypophysitis secondary to initiation of immunotherapy have improved survival outcomes compared to patients who do not [8]. Once again, evidence to support these claims is limited, and the implications on clinical practice guidelines need to be clarified [8, 31].

Less common endocrinopathies, specifically those affecting the pancreatic and adrenal glands, are considered irreversible once they manifest with the initiation of immunotherapy [31]. Long-term management of type 1 diabetes mellitus (T1DM) and primary adrenal insufficiency consists of treatment with insulin therapy and glucocorticoid/mineral corticosteroid therapy, respectively [31]. The prognostic implications of these endocrinopathies on cancer progression and mortality are not well elucidated [8, 31]. However, diabetes mellitus and adrenal insufficiency increase the risk of serious adverse events in patients, such as diabetic ketoacidosis and adrenal crisis, which carry an increased risk of morbidity and mortality [8, 31].

5. Future directions

Cancer immunotherapy has revolutionized the field of oncology, offering a new paradigm in cancer treatment [1]. However, endocrine adverse events (EAEs) have emerged as a significant concern [31]. Ongoing research and clinical trials are crucial in understanding the mechanisms behind these EAEs and developing predictive markers or preventive measures [31].

Current research is focused on understanding the pathophysiology of EAEs [31]. It is hypothesized that immune checkpoint inhibitors may trigger an autoimmune response against endocrine organs, leading to EAEs [31]. Clinical trials are underway to validate this hypothesis and identify the specific antigens targeted by the immune system [21]. In parallel, efforts are being made to identify predictive markers for EAEs [21]. Biomarkers such as autoantibodies, cytokines, and genetic polymorphisms are being investigated for their potential to predict the risk of EAEs [21, 31]. Early identification of patients at risk could allow for proactive management strategies, potentially preventing the onset of EAEs [21, 31]. Several potential biomarkers are being investigated for their ability to predict the risk of EAEs [1, 21].

Circulating blood counts, cytokines, autoantibodies, HLA genotypes, microRNA, gene expression profiling, and serum proteins are among the categories of biomarkers being studied [11]. For instance, certain protein markers such as albumin and thyroid-stimulating hormone are readily accessible in current practice and may serve as potential indicators of EAEs [32]. Autoantibodies are another area of interest. The presence of these antibodies may indicate an autoimmune response against endocrine organs, potentially triggered by immune checkpoint inhibitors, a class of drugs used in immunotherapy [31, 32]. This autoimmune response could lead to EAEs, making autoantibodies a potential predictive marker [32]. Cytokines, small proteins involved in cell signaling, are also being explored as potential biomarkers [32]. Changes in cytokine levels could reflect an immune response to immune checkpoint inhibitors and may be associated with the development of EAEs [32].

While the prediction of EAEs remains a major clinical challenge [21], ongoing research into these and other potential biomarkers holds promise for the early identification and proactive management of EAEs in patients undergoing cancer immunotherapy. As our understanding of these markers improves, so too will our ability to minimize the adverse effects of these revolutionary treatments. Moreover, preventive measures are being explored [31, 32]. One approach is the use of immunosuppressive agents to modulate the immune response [32]. However, this must be balanced against the risk of dampening the anti-tumor effect of immunotherapy [32]. Another strategy is the early detection and management of EAEs through regular monitoring of endocrine function [32].

In conclusion, ongoing research and clinical trials are shedding light on the mechanisms behind EAEs in cancer immunotherapy, paving the way for the development of predictive markers and preventive measures. This will undoubtedly enhance our ability to manage these adverse events, improving patient outcomes in the era of cancer immunotherapy. As we continue to unravel the complexities of the immune system and its interplay with cancer, we move closer to the goal of personalized cancer treatment, maximizing efficacy while minimizing adverse events.

6. Conclusion

Endocrinopathies are common risk factors associated with immune checkpoint inhibitors. Immunotherapy works by stimulating and altering the immune system to detect malignant cells. Most often, PD-L1 and CTLA-4 checkpoint inhibitors may result in the immune system becoming under or overactive, inducing thyroid dysfunction, Adrenal insufficiency, Diabetes Mellitus, and hypophysitis.

Thyroid dysfunction can present as thyroiditis and transition into hypothyroidism (underactive thyroid hormone production) or hyperthyroidism (overactive thyroid hormone production). Monitoring TSH, T4, and T3 (in the case of hyperthyroidism) is essential for thyroid dysfunction management. Treatment of hypothyroidism includes hormone replacement therapy using levothyroxine and beta-blockers for hyperthyroidism. Diagnostic imaging, including thyroid ultrasound and radioactive uptake imaging, can be completed for further thyroid dysfunction detection. Adrenal insufficiency occurs due to either inflammation of the anterior pituitary, as in SAI, or inability of the adrenal gland to produce mineralocorticoids and glucocorticoids, as in PAI. The incidence of the latter is rare and potentially lethal as mineralocorticoids and glucocorticoids are typically essential in the homeostasis of sodium, fluids, and energy, and derangements of these necessary hormones can cause widespread defects. Diagnosis can be made using laboratory tests such as morning draws of cortisol and ACTH, as these are usually high in the morning due to normal circadian rhythms. Morning ACTH, if elevated, is more consistent with PAI, along with decreased serum aldosterone, hyponatremia, and hyperkalemia. Imaging such as head CT and head MRI may elucidate results consistent with enlargement of the pituitary stalk or enhancement of the pituitary gland. Treatment mainly consists of oral corticosteroids, along with fludrocortisone as an additional treatment option in cases of PAI, and thyroid hormone replacement therapy initiated after some time of corticosteroid therapy to mitigate the risk of adrenal crisis. Diabetes Mellitus is less common but life-threatening, with the apparent destruction of T1DM and pancreatic insulin-secreting β-cells.

Diagnostic approaches are centred around diabetes laboratory markers and diagnostic imaging for more severe pancreatic pathologies (pancreatitis). Hypophysitis, induced by CTLA-4 target immunotherapy, results from an inflamed pituitary gland and varies in hormone dysfunction. PD-1/PD-L1-induced hypophysitis targets specific cells known as ACTH-secreting cells found in the pituitary gland. Hypophysitis often presents with generalized symptoms (nausea, vomiting, dizziness, etc.) early in treatment but may become more severe (hypothyroidism, hypogonadism, visual disturbances) when treated with anti-CTLA-4. Laboratory investigations for monitoring of pituitary toxicity include TSH, free T4, morning ACTH and cortisol, prolactin, HbA1C, IGF-1, FSH, LH, and testosterone for males and estradiol for premenopausal females. MRI examination may be completed upon abnormal lab work. The most common treatment for hypophysitis includes holding immunotherapy, beginning steroids or hormone replacement therapy and monitoring.

All management mechanisms should take into consideration patient history and physical examination. Laboratory testing and diagnostic imaging should be used to concrete a diagnosis further. Baseline laboratory should be completed prior to initiating immunotherapy. A summary of endocrinopathies is shown in **Table 1**.

Endocrinopathies	Clinical presentation	Diagnostic approaches	Management Strategies
Thyroid dysfunction	Hypothyroidism [1, 14] • Onset at 71 days with PD-1 & 63 days with combined therapy after initiation Hyperthyroidism [1, 14] • Onset at 47 days with PD-1 & 21 days with combined therapy	Laboratory [15] Hyperthyroidism: decreased TSH, elevated T3, T4 Hypothyroidism: elevated TSH, decreased T3, T4 Diagnostics [15] • Thyroid ultrasound or radioactive thyroid uptake scan	Treatment for hypothyroidism: hormone replacement therapy [2, 11] Symptom management [11] Holding immunotherapy based on symptom severity [1, 14]
Adrenal Insufficiency	Primary adrenal insufficiency [17, 18, 20] • Onset of 119 days after initiation of ICI to symptom Secondary adrenal insufficiency [18] • Onset of 105 days after initiation of ICI to symptom	Laboratory [20] • Low cortisol and elevated ACTH Diagnostics [17, 18, 20] • CT or MRI of the head/ hypophysis	Treatment: corticosteroids. Secondary treatment: thyroid hormone replacement [17, 18, 20] Symptom management [17] Hold/discontinuation of immunotherapy [20]
Diabetes Mellitus	Onset of symptoms between 49 and 119 days after initiation [8]	Laboratory [8, 24] • Elevated plasma glucose, low or absent C-peptide, and mildly elevated glycated hemoglobin (HbA_{1c}) Diagnostics [24] • Not recognized in Canadian diagnostic guidelines	Treatment: monitoring laboratory results and referring to diabetes management team [22] Symptom management [8] Discontinuation of immunotherapy • Grades 3–4 hypercalcemia [22]
Hypophysitis	Onset of symptoms between 42 and 82 days after initiation [27]	Laboratory [27, 28] • TSH, free T4, morning ACTH and cortisol, prolactin, HbA1C, IGF-1, FSH, LH, Testosterone, or estradiol (premenopausal) Diagnostics [23, 27] • Pituitary MRI	Treatment: hormone replacement therapy, glucocorticoids for adrenal crisis [23, 27] Symptom management [25, 31] Holding immunotherapy until symptoms subside [23]

Table 1.
Summary of endocrinopathies.

DOI: http://dx.doi.org/10.5772/intechopen.1004625

Conflict of interest

There are no conflicts of interest to declare.

Author details

Olexiy Aseyev[1,2]*, Alesha Bishop[2], Hannah Shortreed[2], Elycia Monaghan[2] and Yue Sun[2]

1 Thunder Bay Regional Health Science Centre, Thunder Bay, Canada

2 NOSM University, Thunder Bay, Canada

*Address all correspondence to: olexiy.aseyev@tbh.net

References

[1] Esfahani K, Roudaia L, Buhlaiga N, et al. A review of cancer immunotherapy: From the past, to the present, to the future. Current Oncology. 2020;**27**:87-97

[2] Khan M, Maker AV, Jain S. The evolution of cancer immunotherapy. Vaccine. 2021;**9**:1-8. DOI: 10.3390/vaccines9060614 [Epub ahead of print]

[3] Waldman AD, Fritz JM, Lenardo MJ. A guide to cancer immunotherapy: From T cell basic science to clinical practice. Nature Reviews Immunology. 2020;**20**:651-668

[4] Liu C, Yang M, Zhang D, et al. Clinical cancer immunotherapy: Current progress and prospects. Frontiers in Immunology. 2022;**13**:5-8, 15. DOI: 10.3389/fimmu.2022.961805 [Epub ahead of print]

[5] Han Y, Liu D, Li L. PD-1/PD-L1 pathway: Current researches in cancer. 2020. Available from: www.ajcr.us/

[6] Nüssing S, Trapani JA, Parish IA. Revisiting T cell tolerance as a checkpoint target for cancer immunotherapy. Frontiers in Immunology. 2020;**11**:1-7. DOI: 10.3389/fimmu.2020.589641 [Epub ahead of print]

[7] Nogueira E, Newsom-Davis T, Morganstein DL. Immunotherapy-induced endocrinopathies: Assessment, management and monitoring. Therapeutic Advances in Endocrinology and Metabolism. 2019;**10**:1-6. DOI: 10.1177/2042018819896182 [Epub ahead of print]

[8] Hattersley R, Nana M, Lansdown AJ. Endocrine complications of immunotherapies: A review. Clinical Medicine, Journal of the Royal College of Physicians of London. 2021;**21**:E212-E222

[9] Smith DA, Germolec DR. Introduction to immunology and autoimmunity. Environmental Health Perspectives. 1999;**107**(Suppl 5):661-665. DOI: 10.1289/ehp.99107s5661

[10] National Cancer Institute. Immunotherapy to Treat Cancer. NCI; 2019. Available from: https://www.cancer.gov/about-cancer/treatment/types/targeted-therapies

[11] Baraka B, Abosheaishaa H, Nassar M. Immunotherapy-induced thyroid dysfunction: An updated review. The Egyptian Journal of Internal Medicine. 2023;**35**:1-3, 6. DOI: 10.1186/s43162-023-00210-7 [Epub ahead of print]

[12] Buchbinder EI, Desai A. CTLA-4 and PD-1 pathways: Similarities, differences, and implications of their inhibition. American Journal of Clinical Oncology. 2016;**39**:98-106

[13] Brunet-Possenti F, Omgloid V. Immune checkpoint inhibitors-related orchitis. Annals of Oncology. 2017;**28**:906-907

[14] El Sabbagh R, Azar NS, Eid AA, et al. Thyroid dysfunctions due to immune checkpoint inhibitors: A review. International Journal of General Medicine. 2020;**13**:1003-1009

[15] Brahmer JR, Abu-Sbeih H, Ascierto PA, et al. Society for immunotherapy of cancer (sitc) clinical practice guideline on immune checkpoint inhibitor-related adverse events. Journal for ImmunoTherapy of Cancer.

2021;**9**:1-4, 14-15. DOI: 10.1136/jitc-2021-002435 [Epub ahead of print]

[16] Gavrila A. Clinical Thyroidology ® for the Public Development of thyroid problems with immunotherapy drugs for certain cancers is associated with favorable survival. 2020. Available from: https://www.thyroid.org/hypothyroidism/

[17] Cherry G. Immune checkpoint inhibitor-related adrenal insufficiency. Seminars in Oncology Nursing. 2021;**37**(2):1-6. DOI: 10.1016/j.soncn.2021.151131

[18] Cui K, Wang Z, Zhang Q, et al. Immune checkpoint inhibitors and adrenal insufficiency: A large-sample case series study. Annals of Translational Medicine. 2022;**10**:251-251

[19] Martella S, Lucas M, Porcu M, et al. Primary adrenal insufficiency induced by immune checkpoint inhibitors: Biological, clinical, and radiological aspects. Seminars in Oncology. 2023;**22**(52):2-4. DOI: 10.1053/j.seminoncol.2023.11.003 [Epub ahead of print]

[20] Salinas C, Renner A, Rojas C, et al. Primary adrenal insufficiency during immune checkpoint inhibitor treatment: Case reports and review of the literature. Case Reports in Oncology. 2020;**13**:621-626

[21] Kennedy R, Awada H, Vura N, et al. Endocrinopathies from checkpoint inhibitors: Incidence, outcomes, and management. Cleveland Clinic Journal of Medicine. 2023;**90**:307-317

[22] Zheng Z, Liu Y, Yang J, et al. Diabetes mellitus induced by immune checkpoint inhibitors. Diabetes Metabolism Research and Reviews. 2021;**37**(1):2-6. DOI: 10.1002/dmrr.3366

[23] Husebye ES, Castinetti F, Criseno S, et al. Endocrine-related adverse conditions in patients receiving immune checkpoint inhibition: An ESE clinical practice guideline. European Journal of Endocrinology. 2022;**187**:G1-G21

[24] Gauci ML, Laly P, Vidal-Trecan T, et al. Autoimmune diabetes induced by PD-1 inhibitor—Retrospective analysis and pathogenesis: A case report and literature review. Cancer Immunology, Immunotherapy. 2017;**66**:1399-1410

[25] Brahmer JR, Lacchetti C, Schneider BJ, et al. Management of immune-related adverse events in patients treated with immune checkpoint inhibitor therapy: American society of clinical oncology clinical practice guideline. Journal of Clinical Oncology. 2018;**36**:1714-1768

[26] Punthakee Z, Goldenberg R, Katz P. Definition, classification and diagnosis of diabetes, prediabetes and metabolic syndrome. Canadian Journal of Diabetes. 2018;**42**:S10-S15

[27] Prete A, Salvatori R. Hypophysitis. In: Feingold KR, Anawalt B, Blackman MR, et al, editors. Endotext. 2021

[28] Park BC, Jung S, Wright JJ, et al. Recurrence of Hypophysitis after immune checkpoint inhibitor Rechallenge. The Oncologist. 2022;**27**:E967-E969

[29] Özdemir BC. Immune checkpoint inhibitor-related hypogonadism and infertility: A neglected issue in immuno-oncology. Journal for ImmunoTherapy of Cancer. 2021;**9**:1-3. DOI: 10.1136/jitc-2020-002220 [Epub ahead of print]

[30] Izzedine H, Chazal T, Wanchoo R, et al. Immune checkpoint

inhibitor-associated hypercalcaemia. Nephrology Dialysis Transplantation. 2022;**37**:1598-1608

[31] De Filette J, Andreescu CE, Cools F, et al. A systematic review and meta-analysis of endocrine-related adverse events associated with immune checkpoint inhibitors. Hormone and Metabolic Research. 2019;**51**:145-156

[32] Chennamadhavuni A, Abushahin L, Jin N, et al. Risk factors and biomarkers for immune-related adverse events: A practical guide to identifying high-risk patients and rechallenging immune checkpoint inhibitors. Frontiers in Immunology. 2022;**13**:2-4, 9. DOI: 10.3389/fimmu.2022.779691 [Epub ahead of print]

Chapter 7

Challenges and Recent Advances in NK-Mediated Adoptive Cell Therapies against Cancer

Tianxiang Zhang

Abstract

Natural killer (NK) cells play a crucial role in the innate immune system. Unlike adaptive immune cells that rely on specific antigen receptors, NK cell activity is governed by germline-encoded activating or inhibitory receptors expressed on the cell surface. The integration of signals from these receptors determines the NK cell response. Activated NK cells demonstrate potent cytotoxicity against target cells. The distinctive attributes of NK cells, marked by quick response, robust cytotoxicity, and the absence of antigen receptors, position them as promising tools in cancer immunotherapy. Ongoing clinical trials are actively assessing NK cells and related reagents, showing promising outcomes. However, significant challenges arise from the immunosuppressive mechanisms within the tumor microenvironment, impeding the broader application of NK cells. In-depth studies on these mechanisms are imperative to identify solutions, ultimately paving the way for the widespread clinical utilization of NK cells in cancer immunotherapy.

Keywords: nature killer cells, chimera antigen receptor, adoptive cell therapy, tumor immunology, immunotherapy, tumor microenvironment, ADCC

1. Introduction

Natural killer (NK) cells were first described in the 1970s [1–3]. They belong to the innate immune system [4]. More recent studies categorize NK cells as a member of the innate lymphocyte cell (ILC) family [5]. The major site for NK cell development is bone marrow, where NK cells share the same progenitor cells as adaptive immune cells, including both T and B cells [6]. Different from these adaptive immune cells, NK cells do not express antigen receptors but a series of activation or inhibitory receptors that can be triggered by their ligands, usually upregulated or released by viral infected or transformed cells [7–9]. This recognition is quick and, once activated, NK cells can induce apoptosis of target cells without presensitization [1–3]. There are several well-studied activating or inhibitory receptors and pathways governing NK cell activity [7–9]. Among them, the killer Ig-like receptor (KIR) and human leukocyte antigens (HLA) class I axis, or the Ly49 family and major histocompatibility complex (MHC) class I axis in mice, are considered to be the major pathway

IntechOpen

that is involved in NK cell education, mediate the "missing-self" reaction, and inhibit NK cells' activation in normal tissues [9]. The final response of NK cells relies on the integrated signals delivered by all activation and inhibitory signals [9].

During the past several years, adoptive cell therapy (ACT) based cancer immunotherapy has achieved huge success in treating hematopoietic cancers [10]. As a group of robust effector cells, NK has been drawing more and more attention. Compared with T cells, NK cells do not express T-cell receptors and will not induce graft-versus-host disease (GVHD) when applied allogenically [8, 10]. Meanwhile, NK cells can mount a rapid response against target cells in both *in vitro* and *in vivo* studies [1–3]. Indeed, the allogenic application of NK cells was approved to be safe, and the tumor-controlling capability was promising in adult myeloid leukemia patients [11, 12]. Nevertheless, immune suppressive factors, especially in the microenvironment of solid tumors, dampen the efficacy of NK cells, highlighting the importance of deeper mechanism studies [10, 13]. In this chapter, we will review some basic biology of NK cells and how NK cells were applied for cancer treatment, with a focus on the challenges and advances in NK-mediated ACT.

2. The general biology of NK cells

Mature murine NK cells are characterized by signature markers NK1.1+, Nkp46+, and Ly49+, while human NK cells are typically identified as CD3-CD56+ [6]. Unlike adaptive immune cells, NK cells can mature into effector cells independently of the thymus, recombination-activating genes, or activation-induced cytidine deaminase activity [6]. This independence means NK cells lack antigen receptors encoded by rearranged genes, such as the T-cell antigen receptor (TCR) and immunoglobulins [6, 14]. Despite this, NK cells can effectively respond to viral infections or cellular transformation, showcasing various effector functions, notably cytotoxicity and the production of pro-inflammatory cytokines [1–3, 14]. Importantly, NK cell activation does not necessitate prior sensitization, positioning them as sentinel cells integral to immune surveillance [4].

NK cells express a series of activating and inhibitory receptors on the cell surface [9]. The outcome of NK cell activity depends on the result of integrating all the signals received by these receptors (**Figure 1**) [9]. NK cells exhibit versatile mechanisms

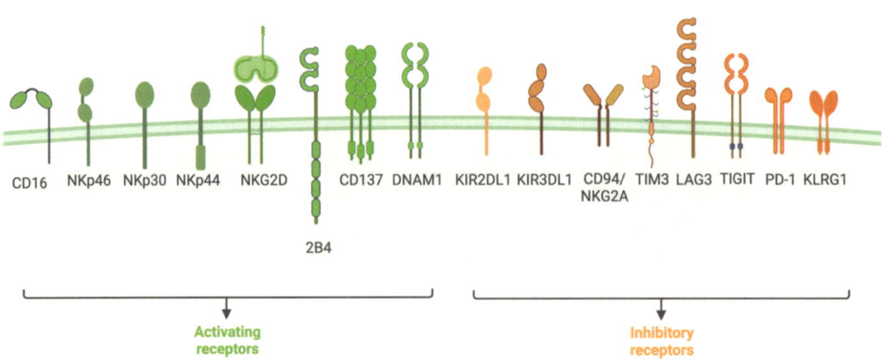

Figure 1.
Activating and inhibitory receptors expressed by human NK cells. Some activating and inhibitory receptors expressed by human NK cells are illustrated. KIR2DL1 and KIR3DL1 were used to represent all KIR2D and KIR3D subfamily members.

in targeting cells, particularly at inflammatory sites guided by chemokine gradients produced by innate or adaptive immune cells [15, 16]. Predominant chemokine-chemokine receptor pathways facilitating NK recruitment include CXCR3–CXCR4, CX3CR1, and CCR3–CCR5 [17]. Upon reaching inflammatory sites, NK cells employ the "missing-self" mechanism, where KIR molecules recognize decreased MHC class I expression on tumor or virally infected cells, relieving inhibitory signals and leading to target cell lysis [9]. Simultaneously, upregulated ligands on these cells bind activating receptors (e.g., NCRs) on NK cell surfaces, initiating natural killing [9]. This unique feature positions NK cells as potential candidates for treating malignancies, evading T-cell recognition and restriction [18].

Another pivotal mechanism in target cell elimination is antibody-dependent cell-mediated cytotoxicity (ADCC). CD16 on NK cell surfaces recognizes the Fc part of antibodies binding to target cells, triggering strong activating signals, degranulation, and target cell lysis [9]. Emerging evidence underscores the significance of ADCC in the clinical success of therapeutic antibodies like rituximab and trastuzumab [19, 20].

Both natural killer activity and ADCC culminate in the release of granzymes and perforin, along with the expression of death ligands such as fas cell surface death receptor ligand (FasL) and tumor necrosis factor-related apoptosis-inducing ligand (TRAIL), inducing cell death [14]. Additionally, NK cells release cytokines, including IFN-γ and TNF-α, contributing to the sustained restriction of target cells [14]. This multifaceted approach highlights the potency of NK cells in combating various cellular threats and underscores their therapeutic potential in addressing malignancies with diverse immune escape strategies.

3. NK-based ACT

In 2013, the cancer-immunity cycle model was introduced as a conceptual framework outlining the functioning of the immune system in regulating tumors [21]. Building on this, the NK cell-cancer cycle model was subsequently proposed, delineating how NK cells exert control over tumor growth (**Figure 2**) [13]. This model delineates several pivotal steps in the process, encompassing the infiltration of NK cells into the tumor lesion, the recognition, and activation of NK cells in response to tumors, the subsequent elimination of tumor cells, and the orchestration of the tumor immune microenvironment [13]. This model offers a comprehensive view of the dynamic interplay between NK cells and cancer, providing insights into the sequential events crucial for NK cells to effectively counteract and manage tumor progression.

The infiltration of NK cells into tumor lesions is a pivotal step in restraining tumor growth, and numerous studies have demonstrated a positive correlation between the abundance and persistence of NK cells in the tumor microenvironment (TME) and increased overall patient survival [22–29]. Chemokines and their corresponding receptors play a crucial role in recruiting NK cells, with $CD56^{dim}$ and $CD56^{bright}$ NK cells in human peripheral blood exhibiting distinct chemokine receptor expression profiles [30]. $CD56^{bright}$ NK cells typically express CCR2, CCR5, CCR7, CXCR3, CXCR4, and CD62L, while $CD56^{dim}$ NK cells express CXCR1, CXCR2, CXCR4, CX3CR1, S1P5, and ChemR23 [10].

Upon entering the TME, NK cells make critical decisions based on the integration of both activating and inhibitory signals. Human NK cells express killer cell immunoglobulin-like receptors (KIRs) that inhibit their activity upon binding to HLA class I molecules expressed on other cells, a mechanism crucial for

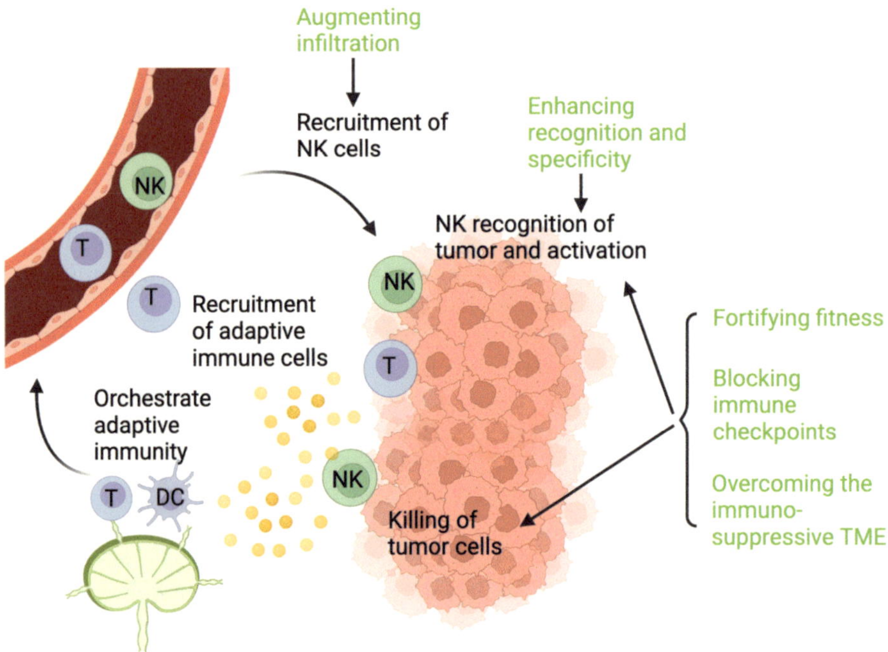

Figure 2.
NK cancer cycle and research priorities dedicated to promoting NK-based immunotherapy (modified from Bald et al. [13]). Once NK cells are recruited to the local tumor lesion, they recognize tumor cells through a series of receptor-ligand interactions. After activation, NK cells kill tumor cells; meanwhile, they release cytokines and chemokines to orchestrate the adaptive immune system and recruit more immune cells to the tumor site. Current research focuses on several aspects, including augmenting infiltration, enhancing recognition and specificity, fortifying NK cells' fitness through cytokines, blocking immune checkpoints, and overcoming the immunosuppressive tumor microenvironment (TME).

self-recognition [9]. Tumor cells, under the adaptive immune system's pressure, often downregulate HLA-I expression, releasing inhibition and lowering the threshold for NK cell activation [31].

Tumor-infiltrating NK cells express activating receptors, including CD16, natural cytotoxicity receptors (NCRs), and NKG2D, which respond to ligands within the TME [7–9, 14, 32]. When activating signals surpass inhibitory ones, NK cells employ multiple mechanisms to secrete effector molecules, inducing tumor cell apoptosis [33, 34]. Activated NK cells also produce pro-inflammatory cytokines, including IFN-γ, GM-CSF, G-CSF, M-CSF, TNF, IL-5, IL-10, and IL-13, reshaping the immune landscape of tumors [14].

Among these cytokines, IFN-γ is one of the best-studied cytokines and plays a multifaceted role in the context of antitumor immune responses [35]. It upregulates the expression of MHC class II and co-stimulatory molecules on antigen-presenting cells and enhances the antigen-processing machinery [36]. It also promotes the non-specific cytocidal activity of macrophages toward tumors [37]. IFN-γ also affects T cells directly. Signaling through IFN-γ in CD4+ T cells can prompt the development of an antitumor TH1 phenotype [38]. This, in turn, leads to an upregulation of granzyme and IL-2 receptor expression on CD8+ T cells, empowering these cells to achieve their maximum cytotoxic potential [35, 39]. IFN-γ stimulates dendritic cells to produce cytokines IL-12 and IL-15 [40]. Together with IFN-γ, these cytokines strongly induce antitumor responses by CD4+ Th1 and cytotoxic CD8+ T cells [41–43]. IFN-γ also augments MHC-I expression on tumor cells, increasing their immunogenicity and susceptibility to recognition by adaptive immune cells [40].

4. Challenges and advances

4.1 Enhance recognition and specificity

The activation of NK cells within tumor lesions is often inadequate due to the heterogeneous and suppressive features of the tumor microenvironment (TME) [10, 13]. Many tumor cells lack sufficient expression of ligands capable of overriding the inhibitory signals delivered by the same cell [44]. Furthermore, in contrast to adaptive immune cells, NK cells do not possess antigen-specific receptors [9]. Consequently, enhancing tumor specificity and improving killing efficacy represent crucial areas garnering considerable research efforts [7, 10, 13, 14].

Chimeric antigen receptors (CARs) are synthetic fusion proteins that combine an extracellular antigen-recognition domain with intracellular signaling moieties to activate cells [10]. Initially tested on T cells, this unique structure delivers potent antigen-specific activation signals to CAR-bearing T cells, leading to substantial clinical success in chimeric antigen receptor T cells (CAR-T) cell therapy [45–51]. Notably, CARs have been successfully adapted for use in generating CAR-NK cells [52, 53]. Clinical trials with a CD19-specific CAR-NK therapy have demonstrated success [54]. Recently, interest has shifted toward designing CARs based on activating signals associated with NK cell biology [55–57]. This includes utilizing adapter proteins like DNAX-activation protein 12 (DAP12) and DAP10 in place of CD3ζ, which has shown efficacy in targeting tumors [57–59].

One critical challenge encountered in the clinical application of CART cell therapy is antigen loss, a phenomenon that contributes to immune evasion by cancer cells [60]. To tackle this challenge, ongoing efforts focus on refining CAR strategies. One approach involves redesigning CARs to target multiple antigens or engage multiple pathways simultaneously [61–63]. The use of dual-CAR or bi-specific CAR designs entails the expression of two different CARs, with each binding to a specific antigen, or incorporating two distinct antigen-recognition domains within a single CAR [61–63]. These designs provide greater flexibility in customization, allowing each CAR to be formatted with both antigen specificity and co-stimulatory signals [61–63].

Enhancing control over CAR-mediated activation is essential to minimize toxicities arising from off-tumor effects [64]. Logic-gated CARs, initially demonstrated in CAR T cells, hold promise for regulating CAR-NK activity [65–69]. Preliminary findings indicate the potential to control CAR-NK activity using logic-gated CAR gene circuits [65–69]. This approach aims to target specific antigens on tumor cells while avoiding interactions with healthy cells [70–72].

Despite the success of CAR-based approaches in targeting surface proteins, a limitation is their inability to detect intracellular antigens [73]. An innovative strategy involves engineering NK cells to express a T-cell receptor (TCR), enabling the recognition of intracellular antigens presented as peptide-HLA complexes [74]. TCR-guided NK-92 cells have demonstrated success in mediating antitumor responses, presenting a potential advantage in avoiding mispairing issues observed in TCR-engineered T cells [74].

NK cell engagers are novel designs that trigger activating receptors on NK cells while binding target antigens on tumor cells [75–79]. Tri-specific and tetra-specific engagers aim to enhance the antitumor effect by targeting multiple antigens or linking cytokines to support NK cell expansion [80–83]. Unlike engineered approaches, engagers bypass gene transfer, offering a simpler and more cost-effective manufacturing process with CAR-like activity [84]. Preclinical studies show promising results in targeting hematologic and solid malignancies [85, 86]. Tri-specific molecules targeting CLEC12A and activating NK cells through engaging CD16 and IL-15 receptors demonstrated a robust response against primary acute myeloid leukemia (AML) blasts [83]. Trifunctional engagers targeting CD16 and NKp46 efficiently controlled tumor growth in solid and metastatic malignancies [87]. Cord blood NK cells complexed with AFM13, a bi-specific engager, exhibited enhanced killing of CD30+ tumor cells, translating to clinical trials for relapsed/refractory CD30+ lymphomas [79]. As strategies advance to clinical trials, assessing the durability of engager-loaded NK cells' antitumor effect and determining the need for multiple treatments become crucial considerations [8].

4.2 Strengthen NK cells' fitness by cytokines

Efforts to enhance NK cell function encompass not only genetic redirection through CAR and TCR engineering but also strategies to prime NK cells *ex vivo* and *in vivo* for sustained antitumor efficacy [88]. The cytolytic capacity of freshly isolated NK cells can be further enhanced by cytokine-mediated activation [89]. *Ex vivo* expansion with IL-2, IL-15, and IL-21 has shown promise in enhancing cytotoxic function, supporting proliferation, and maintaining a nonexhausted state [89]. Another approach involves exposing NK cells to IL-12/15/18, inducing a cytokine-induced memory-like NK cell phenotype that has demonstrated clinical efficacy in patients with relapsed myeloid neoplasias [90, 91]. Additionally, memory-like NK cells engineered with CARs exhibit increased potency against NK-resistant malignancies [92, 93], as observed in clinical trials targeting CD30+ lymphomas with NK cell engagers like AFM13 [79].

While cytokine priming offers advantages, prolonged *ex vivo* stimulation can render NK cells "cytokine-addicted," resulting in decreased persistence without *in vivo* cytokine support [89]. To overcome this challenge, genetic engineering is employed to modify NK cells for autocrine cytokine production, ensuring sustained potency, proliferation, and persistence. CAR-engineered NK cells equipped with additional cytokine signaling, whether released into the environment or in membrane-bound form, exhibit superior persistence in preclinical models [54, 94]. Notably, IL-15-armored CAR-NK cells demonstrated prolonged circulation in patients with CD19+ lymphoid malignancies a year after treatment [54, 94]. These cytokines function not only in a cis manner to enhance NK cells' function but also in a trans manner, inducing a bystander effect that activates other immune effector cells in the tumor microenvironment, potentially amplifying the antitumor response [54, 94]. Optimizing cytokine dosing strategies is crucial for supporting increased function and persistence without inducing metabolic exhaustion [10, 95, 96]. These multifaceted approaches, combining genetic engineering with cytokine modulation, signify a comprehensive strategy to enhance NK cell-based immunotherapies and overcome limitations associated with *ex vivo* stimulation [54, 94–96].

4.3 Blocking immune checkpoints

Tumors employ intricate mechanisms, including immune checkpoint engagement, to evade immune surveillance, potentially restraining NK cells similarly to T cells [10]. Efforts to replicate the clinical success of T-cell checkpoint blockade, such as targeting PD1 and CTLA4, have explored modulating these regulatory circuits in NK cells [97–102]. While some studies suggest their role as functional suppressors, their overall relevance in NK cell biology remains debated [103, 104]. Other regulators like TIM3 [105], TIGIT [106–108], and LAG3 [109] have been investigated, and monoclonal antibody targeting has shown promise in reversing tumor-induced NK dysfunction *in vitro*.

Inhibitory killer cell immunoglobulin-like receptors (KIRs) are potent negative regulators overriding activating signals, attracting interest for their role in suppressing NK cell function. Lirilumab, an anti-panKIR2D antibody, aims to activate NK cells by blocking inhibitory KIRs [110]. However, clinical trials yielded limited success, possibly due to the crucial role of inhibitory KIRs in NK cell education [111, 112]. CD94/NKG2A is another significant NK cell regulator, and monalizumab, disrupting the NKG2A-HLA-E interaction, showed promise in treating recurrent or metastatic squamous cell carcinoma of the head and neck [113].

The current checkpoint-blocking approaches often rely on monoclonal antibodies, requiring multiple infusions due to their limited half-life [114]. Genetic editing advancements allow stable modification of NK cells to regulate mechanisms enhancing effector function [115–117]. For example, disrupting inhibitory receptor NKG2A genetically demonstrated superior tumor control in mouse models [116]. Moreover, genetic engineering targeting CIS (cytokine-inducible SH2-containing protein), a negative regulator of NK cell function, resulted in CAR-NK cells with enhanced metabolic fitness and increased antitumor activity [115, 117].

These studies mentioned above highlight the potential of targeted genetic perturbations to modulate NK cell biology. Moving forward, unbiased high-throughput discovery approaches are expected to systematically elucidate the functional consequences of specific genetic interventions, informing the design of the next generation of NK cell immunotherapies. The convergence of genetic editing capabilities and in-depth functional understanding offers exciting prospects for advancing NK cell-based immunotherapies.

4.4 Overcome immune suppressive TME

The TME presents a challenging metabolic landscape with immunosuppressive features, including glucose and amino acid deprivation, hypoxia, acidity, and an influx of suppressor cells like myeloid-derived suppressor cells (MDSCs) and Tregs [107, 118–135]. In solid tumors, hypoxia is a significant driver of immune cell dysfunction, impairing NK cell function directly and through the presence of immunosuppressive cells [107, 119, 121, 122]. Inhibiting hypoxia-responsive HIF1a signaling in NK cells has been shown to enhance their potency and unleash antitumor function [118].

Tumors exhibit aberrant metabolic behaviors, including high lactic acid levels, nutrient depletion, and increased concentrations of catabolites, adenosine, and reactive oxygen species [120, 128]. To overcome metabolic immunosuppression, current strategies focus on altering tumor metabolism or modifying gene expression in immune cells. Glycolytic inhibitors and lactate dehydrogenase (LDH) blockers show promise, with studies demonstrating improved T-cell antitumor cytotoxicity [124]. Targeting lactate transporters, MCT1 and MCT4, is also under investigation in clinical trials [125]. Adenosine, a by-product of adenosine triphosphate (ATP) metabolism, negatively regulates T-cell and NK cell function in the TME [123, 126, 127, 131]. Strategies to overcome adenosine-mediated immunosuppression include blocking CD73 on tumor cells and genetic editing to delete the adenosine A2A receptor in CAR T cells and CAR-NK cells, showing promise in preclinical studies [129, 134, 136]. Transforming growth factor-beta (TGFβ) signaling is another immunosuppressive mechanism in the TME, adversely affecting NK cell function [133]. Targeted deletion of the TGFβ receptor in NK cells and rendering CB-NK cells immune to TGFβ signaling have demonstrated improved NK cytotoxicity [130, 132, 135].

Given modulating immunometabolism in the TME is a promising direction, striking a balance in modulating immunometabolism is essential, considering that some metabolites are crucial for normal metabolism. Ongoing developments suggest a combined approach involving TME modulation and NK cell engineering could reduce immunosuppression, fostering robust immune cell activity. As these strategies advance, achieving a physiologic balance will be key to optimizing their effectiveness in cancer immunotherapy.

5. Concluding remarks

NK cells have demonstrated significant therapeutic potential in the treatment of AML patients, not only in an autologous context but also through the *ex vivo* differentiation and expansion of NK cells from various sources for allogeneic application. The transfusion of allogeneic NK cells has shown remarkable safety and antitumor efficacy. However, there is still ample room for improvement in overall efficacy, particularly in the treatment of solid tumors. Current research and advancements are concentrated on several facets of the interaction between NK cells and tumor cells. These include, but are not limited to, augmenting infiltration, enhancing recognition and specificity, fortifying NK cells' fitness through cytokines, blocking immune checkpoints, and overcoming the immunosuppressive tumor microenvironment (TME). Genetic modifications have been employed to equip NK cells with chemokines, cytokines, CARs, or TCRs. Multi-specific NK cell engagers are also undergoing active clinical testing. All these approaches are designed to surmount the immunosuppressive challenges posed by the tumor microenvironment and enhance the efficacy of NK-mediated immunotherapies.

In recent times, concerns about safety have arisen in connection with malignancies associated with the genetic manipulation of transferred immune cells [137]. While ongoing discussions primarily center around CAR T cells, it is anticipated that genetically modified NK cells will encounter similar challenges. The use of virus-free methods for gene delivery may mitigate these risks. Furthermore, the *in vivo* editing of lymphocytes and other cells through the application of lipid nanoparticles represents a cutting-edge development in the field of cell and gene therapy [138, 139]. As these technologies progress, new avenues of research are continually unfolding.

Conflict of interest

The authors declare no conflict of interest.

Author details

Tianxiang Zhang
Department of Immunobiology, Yale School of Medicine, Yale University,
New Haven, CT, USA

*Address all correspondence to: tianxiang.zhang@yale.edu

References

[1] Kiessling R, Klein E, Wigzell H. "Natural" killer cells in the mouse. I. Cytotoxic cells with specificity for mouse Moloney leukemia cells. Specificity and distribution according to genotype. European Journal of Immunology. 1975;**5**(2):112-117

[2] Kiessling R, Klein E, Pross H, Wigzell H. "Natural" killer cells in the mouse. II. Cytotoxic cells with specificity for mouse Moloney leukemia cells. Characteristics of the killer cell. European Journal of Immunology. 1975;**5**(2):117-121

[3] Herberman RB, Nunn ME, Holden HT, Lavrin DH. Natural cytotoxic reactivity of mouse lymphoid cells against syngeneic and allogeneic tumors. II. Characterization of effector cells. International Journal of Cancer. 1975;**16**(2):230-239

[4] Vivier E, Raulet DH, Moretta A, Caligiuri MA, Zitvogel L, Lanier LL, et al. Innate or adaptive immunity? The example of natural killer cells. Science. 2011;**331**(6013):44-49

[5] Spits H, Di Santo JP. The expanding family of innate lymphoid cells: Regulators and effectors of immunity and tissue remodeling. Nature Immunology. 2011;**12**(1):21-27

[6] Colucci F, Caligiuri MA, Di Santo JP. What does it take to make a natural killer? Nature Reviews. Immunology. 2003;**3**(5):413-425

[7] Wolf NK, Kissiov DU, Raulet DH. Roles of natural killer cells in immunity to cancer, and applications to immunotherapy. Nature Reviews. Immunology. 2023;**23**(2):90-105

[8] Myers JA, Miller JS. Exploring the NK cell platform for cancer immunotherapy. Nature Reviews. Clinical Oncology. 2021;**18**(2):85-100

[9] Lanier LL. NK cell recognition. Annual Review of Immunology. 2005;**23**:225-274

[10] Laskowski TJ, Biederstadt A, Rezvani K. Natural killer cells in antitumour adoptive cell immunotherapy. Nature Reviews. Cancer. 2022;**22**(10):557-575

[11] Miller JS, Soignier Y, Panoskaltsis-Mortari A, McNearney SA, Yun GH, Fautsch SK, et al. Successful adoptive transfer and in vivo expansion of human haploidentical NK cells in patients with cancer. Blood. 2005;**105**(8):3051-3057

[12] Curti A, Ruggeri L, Parisi S, Bontadini A, Dan E, Motta MR, et al. Larger size of donor alloreactive NK cell repertoire correlates with better response to NK cell immunotherapy in elderly acute myeloid leukemia patients. Clinical Cancer Research. 2016;**22**(8):1914-1921

[13] Bald T, Krummel MF, Smyth MJ, Barry KC. The NK cell-cancer cycle: Advances and new challenges in NK cell-based immunotherapies. Nature Immunology. 2020;**21**(8):835-847

[14] Miller JS, Lanier LL. Natural killer cells in cancer immunotherapy. Annual Review of Cancer Biology. 2019;**3**(1):77-103

[15] Loetscher P, Seitz M, Clark-Lewis I, Baggiolini M, Moser B. Activation of NK cells by CC chemokines. Chemotaxis, Ca2+ mobilization, and enzyme release. Journal of Immunology. 1996;**156**(1):322-327

[16] Maghazachi AA, al-Aoukaty A, Schall TJ. C-C chemokines induce the chemotaxis of NK and IL-2-activated NK cells. Role for G proteins. Journal of Immunology. 1994;**153**(11):4969-4977

[17] Bernardini G, Antonangeli F, Bonanni V, Santoni A. Dysregulation of chemokine/chemokine receptor axes and NK cell tissue localization during diseases. Frontiers in Immunology. 2016;7:402

[18] Malmberg KJ, Sohlberg E, Goodridge JP, Ljunggren HG. Immune selection during tumor checkpoint inhibition therapy paves way for NK-cell "missing self" recognition. Immunogenetics. 2017;**69**(8-9):547-556

[19] Weng WK, Levy R. Two immunoglobulin G fragment C receptor polymorphisms independently predict response to rituximab in patients with follicular lymphoma. Journal of Clinical Oncology. 2003;**21**(21):3940-3947

[20] Varchetta S, Gibelli N, Oliviero B, Nardini E, Gennari R, Gatti G, et al. Elements related to heterogeneity of antibody-dependent cell cytotoxicity in patients under trastuzumab therapy for primary operable breast cancer overexpressing Her2. Cancer Research. 2007;**67**(24):11991-11999

[21] Chen DS, Mellman I. Oncology meets immunology: The cancer-immunity cycle. Immunity. 2013;**39**(1):1-10

[22] Wu M, Mei F, Liu W, Jiang J. Comprehensive characterization of tumor infiltrating natural killer cells and clinical significance in hepatocellular carcinoma based on gene expression profiles. Biomedicine & Pharmacotherapy. 2020;**121**:109637

[23] Barry KC, Hsu J, Broz ML, Cueto FJ, Binnewies M, Combes AJ, et al. A natural killer-dendritic cell axis defines checkpoint therapy-responsive tumor microenvironments. Nature Medicine. 2018;**24**(8):1178-1191

[24] Bottcher JP, Bonavita E, Chakravarty P, Blees H, Cabeza-Cabrerizo M, Sammicheli S, et al. NK cells stimulate recruitment of cDC1 into the tumor microenvironment promoting cancer immune control. Cell. 2018;**172**(5):1022-1037.e14

[25] Takanami I, Takeuchi K, Giga M. The prognostic value of natural killer cell infiltration in resected pulmonary adenocarcinoma. The Journal of Thoracic and Cardiovascular Surgery. 2001;**121**(6):1058-1063

[26] Ishigami S, Natsugoe S, Tokuda K, Nakajo A, Che X, Iwashige H, et al. Prognostic value of intratumoral natural killer cells in gastric carcinoma. Cancer. 2000;**88**(3):577-583

[27] Villegas FR, Coca S, Villarrubia VG, Jimenez R, Chillon MJ, Jareno J, et al. Prognostic significance of tumor infiltrating natural killer cells subset CD57 in patients with squamous cell lung cancer. Lung Cancer. 2002;**35**(1):23-28

[28] Muntasell A, Rojo F, Servitja S, Rubio-Perez C, Cabo M, Tamborero D, et al. NK cell infiltrates and HLA class I expression in primary HER2(+) breast cancer predict and uncouple pathological response and disease-free survival. Clinical Cancer Research. 2019;**25**(5):1535-1545

[29] Remark R, Alifano M, Cremer I, Lupo A, Dieu-Nosjean MC, Riquet M, et al. Characteristics and clinical impacts of the immune environments in colorectal and renal cell carcinoma lung metastases: Influence of tumor origin. Clinical Cancer Research. 2013;**19**(15):4079-4091

[30] Melsen JE, Lugthart G, Lankester AC, Schilham MW. Human circulating and tissue-resident CD56(bright) natural killer cell populations. Frontiers in Immunology. 2016;**7**:262

[31] Hicklin DJ, Marincola FM, Ferrone S. HLA class I antigen downregulation in human cancers: T-cell immunotherapy revives an old story. Molecular Medicine Today. 1999;**5**(4):178-186

[32] Reina-Ortiz C, Giraldos D, Azaceta G, Palomera L, Marzo I, Naval J, et al. Harnessing the potential of NK cell-based immunotherapies against multiple myeloma. Cells. 2022;**11**(3):392

[33] Browne KA, Blink E, Sutton VR, Froelich CJ, Jans DA, Trapani JA. Cytosolic delivery of granzyme B by bacterial toxins: Evidence that endosomal disruption, in addition to transmembrane pore formation, is an important function of perforin. Molecular and Cellular Biology. 1999;**19**(12):8604-8615

[34] Smyth MJ, Cretney E, Kelly JM, Westwood JA, Street SE, Yagita H, et al. Activation of NK cell cytotoxicity. Molecular Immunology. 2005;**42**(4):501-510

[35] Alspach E, Lussier DM, Schreiber RD. Interferon gamma and its important roles in promoting and inhibiting spontaneous and therapeutic cancer immunity. Cold Spring Harbor Perspectives in Biology. 2019;**11**(3):a028480

[36] Pan J, Zhang M, Wang J, Wang Q, Xia D, Sun W, et al. Interferon-gamma is an autocrine mediator for dendritic cell maturation. Immunology Letters. 2004;**94**(1-2):141-151

[37] Shapouri-Moghaddam A, Mohammadian S, Vazini H, Taghadosi M, Esmaeili SA, Mardani F, et al. Macrophage plasticity, polarization, and function in health and disease. Journal of Cellular Physiology. 2018;**233**(9): 6425-6440

[38] Bradley LM, Dalton DK, Croft M. A direct role for IFN-gamma in regulation of Th1 cell development. Journal of Immunology. 1996;**157**(4):1350-1358

[39] Burke JD, Young HA. IFN-gamma: A cytokine at the right time, is in the right place. Seminars in Immunology. 2019;**43**:101280

[40] Jorgovanovic D, Song M, Wang L, Zhang Y. Roles of IFN-gamma in tumor progression and regression: A review. Biomarker Research. 2020;**8**:49

[41] Kelly JM, Darcy PK, Markby JL, Godfrey DI, Takeda K, Yagita H, et al. Induction of tumor-specific T cell memory by NK cell-mediated tumor rejection. Nature Immunology. 2002;**3**(1):83-90

[42] Cerwenka A, Baron JL, Lanier LL. Ectopic expression of retinoic acid early inducible-1 gene (RAE-1) permits natural killer cell-mediated rejection of a MHC class I-bearing tumor in vivo. Proceedings of the National Academy of Sciences of the United States of America. 2001;**98**(20):11521-11526

[43] Mocikat R, Braumuller H, Gumy A, Egeter O, Ziegler H, Reusch U, et al. Natural killer cells activated by MHC class I(low) targets prime dendritic cells to induce protective CD8 T cell responses. Immunity. 2003;**19**(4):561-569

[44] Vitale M, Cantoni C, Pietra G, Mingari MC, Moretta L. Effect of tumor cells and tumor microenvironment on NK-cell function. European Journal of Immunology. 2014;**44**(6):1582-1592

[45] Maude SL, Laetsch TW, Buechner J, Rives S, Boyer M, Bittencourt H, et al. Tisagenlecleucel in children and young adults with B-cell lymphoblastic leukemia. The New England Journal of Medicine. 2018;**378**(5):439-448

[46] Schuster SJ, Bishop MR, Tam CS, Waller EK, Borchmann P, McGuirk JP, et al. Tisagenlecleucel in adult relapsed or refractory diffuse large B-cell lymphoma. The New England Journal of Medicine. 2019;**380**(1):45-56

[47] Neelapu SS, Locke FL, Bartlett NL, Lekakis LJ, Miklos DB, Jacobson CA, et al. Axicabtagene ciloleucel CAR T-cell therapy in refractory large B-cell lymphoma. The New England Journal of Medicine. 2017;**377**(26):2531-2544

[48] Park JH, Riviere I, Gonen M, Wang X, Senechal B, Curran KJ, et al. Long-term follow-up of CD19 CAR therapy in acute lymphoblastic leukemia. The New England Journal of Medicine. 2018;**378**(5):449-459

[49] Wang M, Munoz J, Goy A, Locke FL, Jacobson CA, Hill BT, et al. KTE-X19 CAR T-cell therapy in relapsed or refractory mantle-cell lymphoma. The New England Journal of Medicine. 2020;**382**(14):1331-1342

[50] Munshi NC, Anderson LD Jr, Shah N, Madduri D, Berdeja J, Lonial S, et al. Idecabtagene vicleucel in relapsed and refractory multiple myeloma. The New England Journal of Medicine. 2021;**384**(8):705-716

[51] Raje N, Berdeja J, Lin Y, Siegel D, Jagannath S, Madduri D, et al. Anti-BCMA CAR T-cell therapy bb2121 in relapsed or refractory multiple myeloma. The New England Journal of Medicine. 2019;**380**(18):1726-1737

[52] Biederstadt A, Rezvani K. Engineering the next generation of CAR-NK immunotherapies. International Journal of Hematology. 2021;**114**(5):554-571

[53] Daher M, Rezvani K. Outlook for new CAR-based therapies with a focus on CAR NK cells: What lies beyond CAR-engineered T cells in the race against cancer. Cancer Discovery. 2021;**11**(1):45-58

[54] Liu E, Marin D, Banerjee P, Macapinlac HA, Thompson P, Basar R, et al. Use of CAR-transduced natural killer cells in CD19-positive lymphoid tumors. The New England Journal of Medicine. 2020;**382**(6):545-553

[55] Zhao R, Cheng L, Jiang Z, Wei X, Li B, Wu Q, et al. DNAX-activating protein 10 co-stimulation enhances the anti-tumor efficacy of chimeric antigen receptor T cells. Oncoimmunology. 2019;**8**(1):e1509173

[56] Ng YY, Tay JCK, Li Z, Wang J, Zhu J, Wang S. T cells expressing NKG2D CAR with a DAP12 signaling domain stimulate lower cytokine production while effective in tumor eradication. Molecular Therapy. 2021;**29**(1):75-85

[57] Billadeau DD, Upshaw JL, Schoon RA, Dick CJ, Leibson PJ. NKG2D-DAP10 triggers human NK cell-mediated killing via a Syk-independent regulatory pathway. Nature Immunology. 2003;**4**(6):557-564

[58] Lanier LL, Corliss BC, Wu J, Leong C, Phillips JH. Immunoreceptor DAP12 bearing a tyrosine-based activation motif is involved in activating NK cells. Nature. 1998;**391**(6668):703-707

[59] Topfer K, Cartellieri M, Michen S, Wiedemuth R, Muller N, Lindemann D,

et al. DAP12-based activating chimeric antigen receptor for NK cell tumor immunotherapy. Journal of Immunology. 2015;**194**(7):3201-3212

[60] Johnson GA, Locke FL. Mechanisms of resistance to chimeric antigen receptor T cell therapy. Hematology/Oncology Clinics of North America. 2023;**37**(6):1189-1199

[61] Cronk RJ, Zurko J, Shah NN. Bispecific chimeric antigen receptor T cell therapy for B cell malignancies and multiple myeloma. Cancers (Basel). 2020;**12**(9):2523

[62] Shah NN, Johnson BD, Schneider D, Zhu F, Szabo A, Keever-Taylor CA, et al. Bispecific anti-CD20, anti-CD19 CAR T cells for relapsed B cell malignancies: A phase 1 dose escalation and expansion trial. Nature Medicine. 2020;**26**(10):1569-1575

[63] Zah E, Nam E, Bhuvan V, Tran U, Ji BY, Gosliner SB, et al. Systematically optimized BCMA/CS1 bispecific CAR-T cells robustly control heterogeneous multiple myeloma. Nature Communications. 2020;**11**(1):2283

[64] Rafiq S, Hackett CS, Brentjens RJ. Engineering strategies to overcome the current roadblocks in CAR T cell therapy. Nature Reviews. Clinical Oncology. 2020;**17**(3):147-167

[65] Gonzalez A, Roguev A, Frankel NW, Garrison BS, Lee D, Gainer M, et al. Development of logic-gated CAR-NK cells to reduce target-mediated healthy tissue toxicities. Cancer Research. 2021;**81**(13):LB028

[66] Muftuoglu M, Basyal M, Li L, Lv JX, Ostermann LB, Zhao R, et al. Calibrated release IL15 bivalent CD33 and/or FLT3 and NOT Emcn logic gated gene circuit CAR-NK cell therapy (SENTI-202) in venetoclax resistant patient derived xenograft acute myeloid leukemia models. Blood. 2023;**142**(Suppl. 1): 4831

[67] Gonzalez A, Hong EP, Yucel G, Leitner E, Chinta P, Deng H, et al. Preclinical development of SENTI-202, an off-the-shelf logic gated CAR-NK cell therapy, for the treatment of CD33/FLT3+hematologic malignancies including AML. Cancer Research. 2023;**83**(Suppl. 7):3195

[68] Junca AG, Frankel N, Morvan M, Roguev A, Hung M, Gordley R, et al. Senti-401, an allogeneic logic-gated and multiarmed Car-Nk cell therapy for the treatment of Cea-expressing solid tumors with enhanced selectivity and efficacy, journal for immunotherapy of. Cancer. 2022;**10**:A235-A235

[69] Garrison B, Deng H, Yucel G, Frankel N, Gordley R, Hung M, et al. Logic gated FLT3 or CD33 not EMCN CAR-NK cell therapy (SENTI-202) for precise targeting of AML. Molecular Therapy. 2022;**30**(4):398-399

[70] Wallstabe L, Gottlich C, Nelke LC, Kuhnemundt J, Schwarz T, Nerreter T, et al. ROR1-CAR T cells are effective against lung and breast cancer in advanced microphysiologic 3D tumor models. JCI Insight. 2019;**4**(18):e126345

[71] Srivastava S, Salter AI, Liggitt D, Yechan-Gunja S, Sarvothama M, Cooper K, et al. Logic-gated ROR1 chimeric antigen receptor expression rescues T cell-mediated toxicity to normal tissues and enables selective tumor targeting. Cancer Cell. 2019;**35**(3):489-503.e8

[72] Cho JH, Okuma A, Sofjan K, Lee S, Collins JJ, Wong WW. Engineering advanced logic and distributed computing in human CAR immune

cells. Nature Communications. 2021;**12**(1):792

[73] Sterner RC, Sterner RM. CAR-T cell therapy: Current limitations and potential strategies. Blood Cancer Journal. 2021;**11**(4):69

[74] Mensali N, Dillard P, Hebeisen M, Lorenz S, Theodossiou T, Myhre MR, et al. NK cells specifically TCR-dressed to kill cancer cells. eBioMedicine. 2019;**40**:106-117

[75] Wiernik A, Foley B, Zhang B, Verneris MR, Warlick E, Gleason MK, et al. Targeting natural killer cells to acute myeloid leukemia in vitro with a CD16 x 33 bispecific killer cell engager and ADAM17 inhibition. Clinical Cancer Research. 2013;**19**(14):3844-3855

[76] Vallera DA, Zhang B, Gleason MK, Oh S, Weiner LM, Kaufman DS, et al. Heterodimeric bispecific single-chain variable-fragment antibodies against EpCAM and CD16 induce effective antibody-dependent cellular cytotoxicity against human carcinoma cells. Cancer Biotherapy & Radiopharmaceuticals. 2013;**28**(4):274-282

[77] Gleason MK, Ross JA, Warlick ED, Lund TC, Verneris MR, Wiernik A, et al. CD16xCD33 bispecific killer cell engager (BiKE) activates NK cells against primary MDS and MDSC CD33+ targets. Blood. 2014;**123**(19):3016-3026

[78] Schmohl JU, Gleason MK, Dougherty PR, Miller JS, Vallera DA. Heterodimeric bispecific single chain variable fragments (scFv) killer engagers (BiKEs) enhance NK-cell activity against CD133+ colorectal cancer cells. Targeted Oncology. 2016;**11**(3):353-361

[79] Kerbauy LN, Marin ND, Kaplan M, Banerjee PP, Berrien-Elliott MM, Becker-Hapak M, et al. Combining AFM13, a bispecific CD30/CD16 antibody, with cytokine-activated blood and cord blood-derived NK cells facilitates CAR-like responses against CD30(+) malignancies. Clinical Cancer Research. 2021;**27**(13):3744-3756

[80] Reusch U, Burkhardt C, Fucek I, Le Gall F, Le Gall M, Hoffmann K, et al. A novel tetravalent bispecific TandAb (CD30/CD16A) efficiently recruits NK cells for the lysis of CD30+ tumor cells. MAbs. 2014;**6**(3):728-739

[81] Vallera DA, Felices M, McElmurry R, McCullar V, Zhou X, Schmohl JU, et al. IL15 trispecific killer engagers (TriKE) make natural killer cells specific to CD33+ targets while also inducing persistence, in vivo expansion, and enhanced function. Clinical Cancer Research. 2016;**22**(14):3440-3450

[82] Schmohl JU, Felices M, Oh F, Lenvik AJ, Lebeau AM, Panyam J, et al. Engineering of anti-CD133 trispecific molecule capable of inducing NK expansion and driving antibody-dependent cell-mediated cytotoxicity. Cancer Research and Treatment. 2017;**49**(4):1140-1152

[83] Arvindam US, van Hauten PMM, Schirm D, Schaap N, Hobo W, Blazar BR, et al. A trispecific killer engager molecule against CLEC12A effectively induces NK-cell mediated killing of AML cells. Leukemia. 2021;**35**(6):1586-1596

[84] Goebeler ME, Bargou RC. T cell-engaging therapies—BiTEs and beyond. Nature Reviews. Clinical Oncology. 2020;**17**(7):418-434

[85] Hibler W, Merlino G, Yu Y. CAR NK cell therapy for the treatment of metastatic melanoma: Potential & prospects. Cells. 2023;**12**(23):2750

[86] Fetzko SL, Timothy LD, Parihar R. NK cell therapeutics for hematologic malignancies: From potential to fruition. Current Hematologic Malignancy Reports. 2023;**18**(6):264-272

[87] Gauthier L, Morel A, Anceriz N, Rossi B, Blanchard-Alvarez A, Grondin G, et al. Multifunctional natural killer cell engagers targeting NKp46 trigger protective tumor immunity. Cell. 2019;**177**(7):1701-1713.e16

[88] Granzin M, Wagner J, Kohl U, Cerwenka A, Huppert V, Ullrich E. Shaping of natural killer cell antitumor activity by ex vivo cultivation. Frontiers in Immunology. 2017;**8**:458

[89] Miller JS. Therapeutic applications: Natural killer cells in the clinic. Hematology. American Society of Hematology. Education Program. 2013;**2013**:247-253

[90] Romee R, Rosario M, Berrien-Elliott MM, Wagner JA, Jewell BA, Schappe T, et al. Cytokine-induced memory-like natural killer cells exhibit enhanced responses against myeloid leukemia. Science Translational Medicine. 2016;**8**(357):357ra123

[91] Shapiro RM, Birch GC, Hu G, Vergara Cadavid J, Nikiforow S, Baginska J, et al. Expansion, persistence, and efficacy of donor memory-like NK cells infused for posttransplant relapse. The Journal of Clinical Investigation. 2022;**132**(11):e154334

[92] Gang M, Marin ND, Wong P, Neal CC, Marsala L, Foster M, et al. CAR-modified memory-like NK cells exhibit potent responses to NK-resistant lymphomas. Blood. 2020;**136**(20):2308-2318

[93] Dong H, Xie G, Liang Y, Ham JD, Vergara J, Chen J, et al. Engineered memory-like NK cars targeting a neoepitope derived from intracellular NPM1c exhibit potent activity and specificity against acute myeloid leukemia. Blood. 2020;**136**(Suppl. 1):3

[94] Liu E, Tong Y, Dotti G, Shaim H, Savoldo B, Mukherjee M, et al. Cord blood NK cells engineered to express IL-15 and a CD19-targeted CAR show long-term persistence and potent antitumor activity. Leukemia. 2018;**32**(2):520-531

[95] Lopez-Cantillo G, Uruena C, Camacho BA, Ramirez-Segura C. CAR-T cell performance: How to improve their persistence? Frontiers in Immunology. 2022;**13**:878209

[96] Shen L, Xiao Y, Tian J, Lu Z. Remodeling metabolic fitness: Strategies for improving the efficacy of chimeric antigen receptor T cell therapy. Cancer Letters. 2022;**529**:139-152

[97] Stojanovic A, Fiegler N, Brunner-Weinzierl M, Cerwenka A. CTLA-4 is expressed by activated mouse NK cells and inhibits NK cell IFN-gamma production in response to mature dendritic cells. Journal of Immunology. 2014;**192**(9):4184-4191

[98] Sanseviero E, O'Brien EM, Karras JR, Shabaneh TB, Aksoy BA, Xu W, et al. Anti-CTLA-4 activates intratumoral NK cells and combined with IL15/IL15Ralpha complexes enhances tumor control. Cancer Immunology Research. 2019;**7**(8):1371-1380

[99] Judge SJ, Dunai C, Aguilar EG, Vick SC, Sturgill IR, Khuat LT, et al. Minimal PD-1 expression in mouse and human NK cells under diverse conditions. The Journal of Clinical Investigation. 2020;**130**(6):3051-3068

[100] Davis Z, Felices M, Lenvik T, Badal S, Walker JT, Hinderlie P, et al. Low-density PD-1 expression on resting human natural killer cells is functional and upregulated after transplantation. Blood Advances. 2021;**5**(4):1069-1080

[101] Hsu J, Hodgins JJ, Marathe M, Nicolai CJ, Bourgeois-Daigneault MC, Trevino TN, et al. Contribution of NK cells to immunotherapy mediated by PD-1/PD-L1 blockade. The Journal of Clinical Investigation. 2018;**128**(10): 4654-4668

[102] Dong W, Wu X, Ma S, Wang Y, Nalin AP, Zhu Z, et al. The mechanism of anti-PD-L1 antibody efficacy against PD-L1-negative tumors identifies NK cells expressing PD-L1 as a cytolytic effector. Cancer Discovery. 2019;**9**(10):1422-1437

[103] Newman J, Horowitz A. NK cells seize PD1 from leukaemia cells. Nature Reviews. Immunology. 2021;**21**(6):345

[104] Judge SJ, Murphy WJ, Canter RJ. Characterizing the dysfunctional NK cell: Assessing the clinical relevance of exhaustion, anergy, and senescence. Frontiers in Cellular and Infection Microbiology. 2020;**10**:49

[105] da Silva IP, Gallois A, Jimenez-Baranda S, Khan S, Anderson AC, Kuchroo VK, et al. Reversal of NK-cell exhaustion in advanced melanoma by Tim-3 blockade. Cancer Immunology Research. 2014;**2**(5):410-422

[106] Chauvin JM, Ka M, Pagliano O, Menna C, Ding Q, DeBlasio R, et al. IL15 stimulation with TIGIT blockade reverses CD155-mediated NK-cell dysfunction in melanoma. Clinical Cancer Research. 2020;**26**(20):5520-5533

[107] Sarhan D, Hippen KL, Lemire A, Hying S, Luo X, Lenvik T, et al. Adaptive NK cells resist regulatory T-cell suppression driven by IL37. Cancer Immunology Research. 2018;**6**(7):766-775

[108] Zhang Q, Bi J, Zheng X, Chen Y, Wang H, Wu W, et al. Blockade of the checkpoint receptor TIGIT prevents NK cell exhaustion and elicits potent anti-tumor immunity. Nature Immunology. 2018;**19**(7):723-732

[109] Ali AM, Moran MT, Tuazon J, Gyurova I, Vignali DAA, Waggoner SN. LAG-3 modulation of natural killer cell immunoregulatory function. Journal of Immunology. 2019;**202**(1_Supplement):7

[110] Kohrt HE, Thielens A, Marabelle A, Sagiv-Barfi I, Sola C, Chanuc F, et al. Anti-KIR antibody enhancement of anti-lymphoma activity of natural killer cells as monotherapy and in combination with anti-CD20 antibodies. Blood. 2014;**123**(5):678-686

[111] Vey M, Dumas PY, Recher C, Gastaud L, Lioure B, Bulabois CE, et al. Randomized phase 2 trial of Lirilumab (anti-KIR monoclonal antibody, mAb) as maintenance treatment in elderly patients (pts) with acute myeloid leukemia (AML): Results of the Effikir trial. Blood. 2017;**130**(Suppl. 1):889

[112] Vey N, Karlin L, Sadot-Lebouvier S, Broussais F, Berton-Rigaud D, Rey J, et al. A phase 1 study of lirilumab (antibody against killer immunoglobulin-like receptor antibody KIR2D; IPH2102) in patients with solid tumors and hematologic malignancies. Oncotarget. 2018;**9**(25):17675-17688

[113] Andre P, Denis C, Soulas C, Bourbon-Caillet C, Lopez J, Arnoux T, et al. Anti-NKG2A mAb is a checkpoint inhibitor that promotes anti-tumor immunity by unleashing both T and NK cells. Cell. 2018;**175**(7):1731-1743.e13

[114] Chames P, Van Regenmortel M, Weiss E, Baty D. Therapeutic antibodies: Successes, limitations and hopes for the future. British Journal of Pharmacology. 2009;**157**(2):220-233

[115] Daher M, Basar R, Gokdemir E, Baran N, Uprety N, Nunez Cortes AK, et al. Targeting a cytokine checkpoint enhances the fitness of armored cord blood CAR-NK cells. Blood. 2021;**137**(5):624-636

[116] Kamiya T, Seow SV, Wong D, Robinson M, Campana D. Blocking expression of inhibitory receptor NKG2A overcomes tumor resistance to NK cells. The Journal of Clinical Investigation. 2019;**129**(5):2094-2106

[117] Zhu H, Blum RH, Bernareggi D, Ask EH, Wu Z, Hoel HJ, et al. Metabolic reprograming via deletion of CISH in human iPSC-derived NK cells promotes in vivo persistence and enhances anti-tumor activity. Cell Stem Cell. 2020;**27**(2):224-237.e6

[118] Ni J, Wang X, Stojanovic A, Zhang Q, Wincher M, Buhler L, et al. Single-cell RNA sequencing of tumor-infiltrating NK cells reveals that inhibition of transcription factor HIF-1alpha unleashes NK cell activity. Immunity. 2020;**52**(6):1075-1087.e8

[119] Nunez SY, Ziblat A, Secchiari F, Torres NI, Sierra JM, Raffo Iraolagoitia XL, et al. Human M2 macrophages limit NK cell effector functions through secretion of TGF-beta and engagement of CD85j. Journal of Immunology. 2018;**200**(3):1008-1015

[120] Renner K, Singer K, Koehl GE, Geissler EK, Peter K, Siska PJ, et al. Metabolic hallmarks of tumor and immune cells in the tumor microenvironment. Frontiers in Immunology. 2017;**8**:248

[121] Tumino N, Di Pace AL, Besi F, Quatrini L, Vacca P, Moretta L. Interaction between MDSC and NK cells in solid and hematological malignancies: Impact on HSCT. Frontiers in Immunology. 2021;**12**:638841

[122] Zalfa C, Paust S. Natural killer cell interactions with myeloid derived suppressor cells in the tumor microenvironment and implications for cancer immunotherapy. Frontiers in Immunology. 2021;**12**:633205

[123] Allard B, Longhi MS, Robson SC, Stagg J. The ectonucleotidases CD39 and CD73: Novel checkpoint inhibitor targets. Immunological Reviews. 2017;**276**(1):121-144

[124] Cascone T, McKenzie JA, Mbofung RM, Punt S, Wang Z, Xu C, et al. Increased tumor glycolysis characterizes immune resistance to adoptive T cell therapy. Cell Metabolism. 2018;**27**(5):977-987.e4

[125] Halford S, Veal GJ, Wedge SR, Payne GS, Bacon CM, Sloan P, et al. A phase I dose-escalation study of AZD3965, an oral monocarboxylate transporter 1 inhibitor, in patients with advanced cancer. Clinical Cancer Research. 2023;**29**(8):1429-1439

[126] Jin D, Fan J, Wang L, Thompson LF, Liu A, Daniel BJ, et al. CD73 on tumor cells impairs antitumor T-cell responses: A novel mechanism of tumor-induced immune suppression. Cancer Research. 2010;**70**(6):2245-2255

[127] Stagg J, Divisekera U, McLaughlin N, Sharkey J, Pommey S, Denoyer D, et al. Anti-CD73 antibody therapy inhibits breast tumor growth and metastasis. Proceedings of the National Academy of Sciences of the United States of America. 2010;**107**(4):1547-1552

[128] Wei F, Wang D, Wei J, Tang N, Tang L, Xiong F, et al. Metabolic crosstalk in the tumor microenvironment regulates antitumor immunosuppression and immunotherapy resisitance. Cellular and Molecular Life Sciences. 2021;**78**(1):173-193

[129] Giuffrida L, Sek K, Henderson MA, Lai J, Chen AXY, Meyran D, et al. CRISPR/Cas9 mediated deletion of the adenosine A2A receptor enhances CAR T cell efficacy. Nature Communications. 2021;**12**(1):3236

[130] Kim TD, Lee SU, Yun S, Sun HN, Lee SH, Kim JW, et al. Human microRNA-27a* targets Prf1 and GzmB expression to regulate NK-cell cytotoxicity. Blood. 2011;**118**(20):5476-5486

[131] Perrot I, Michaud HA, Giraudon-Paoli M, Augier S, Docquier A, Gros L, et al. Blocking antibodies targeting the CD39/CD73 immunosuppressive pathway unleash immune responses in combination cancer therapies. Cell Reports. 2019;**27**(8):2411-2425.e9

[132] Shaim H, Shanley M, Basar R, Daher M, Gumin J, Zamler DB, et al. Targeting the alphav integrin/TGF-beta axis improves natural killer cell function against glioblastoma stem cells. The Journal of Clinical Investigation. 2021;**131**(14):e142116

[133] Viel S, Marcais A, Guimaraes FS, Loftus R, Rabilloud J, Grau M, et al. TGF-beta inhibits the activation and functions of NK cells by repressing the mTOR pathway. Science Signaling. 2016;**9**(415):ra19

[134] Young A, Ngiow SF, Gao Y, Patch AM, Barkauskas DS, Messaoudene M, et al. A2AR adenosine signaling suppresses natural killer cell maturation in the tumor microenvironment. Cancer Research. 2018;**78**(4):1003-1016

[135] Yvon ES, Burga R, Powell A, Cruz CR, Fernandes R, Barese C, et al. Cord blood natural killer cells expressing a dominant negative TGF-beta receptor: Implications for adoptive immunotherapy for glioblastoma. Cytotherapy. 2017;**19**(3):408-418

[136] Young A, Ngiow SF, Barkauskas DS, Sult E, Hay C, Blake SJ, et al. Co-inhibition of CD73 and A2AR adenosine signaling improves anti-tumor immune responses. Cancer Cell. 2016;**30**(3):391-403

[137] Micklethwaite KP, Gowrishankar K, Gloss BS, Li Z, Street JA, Moezzi L, et al. Investigation of product-derived lymphoma following infusion of piggyBac-modified CD19 chimeric antigen receptor T cells. Blood. 2021;**138**(16):1391-1405

[138] Aghajanian H, Kimura T, Rurik JG, Hancock AS, Leibowitz MS, Li L, et al. Targeting cardiac fibrosis with engineered T cells. Nature. 2019;**573**(7774):430-433

[139] Rurik JG, Tombacz I, Yadegari A, Mendez Fernandez PO, Shewale SV, Li L, et al. CAR T cells produced in vivo to treat cardiac injury. Science. 2022;**375**(6576):91-96